Advancing Occupational Therapy in Mental Health Practice

Dedication

This book is dedicated to the memory of the late Hester Monteath, MBE, D.Ed, FCOT a pioneering occupational therapist whose vision, courage and determination benefited people with mental health problems. Furthermore, she inspired generations of occupational therapists to specialise in mental health practice – her spirit lives on.

Advancing Occupational Therapy in Mental Health Practice

Edited by

Elizabeth Anne McKay

Christine Craik

Kee Hean Lim

and

Gabrielle Richards

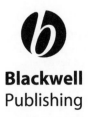

Blackwell
Publishing

© 2008 by Blackwell Publishing Ltd

Blackwell Publishing editorial offices:
Blackwell Publishing Ltd, 9600 Garsington Road, Oxford OX4 2DQ, UK
  Tel: +44 (0)1865 776868
Blackwell Publishing Inc., 350 Main Street, Malden, MA 02148-5020, USA
  Tel: +1 781 388 8250
Blackwell Publishing Asia Pty Ltd, 550 Swanston Street, Carlton, Victoria 3053, Australia
  Tel: +61 (0)3 8359 1011

First published 2008 by Blackwell Publishing Ltd

ISBN: 978-1-4051-5852-7

Library of Congress Cataloging-in-Publication Data

Advancing occupational therapy in mental health practice / edited by Elizabeth Anne McKay ... [et al.].
    p. ; cm.
Includes bibliographical references and index.
    ISBN-13: 978-1-4051-5852-7 (pbk. : alk. paper)
    ISBN-10: 1-4051-5852-2 (pbk. : alk. paper) 1. Occupational therapy. 2. Mentally ill–Rehabilitation.
I. McKay, Elizabeth Anne.
[DNLM: 1. Mental Health Services–trends. 2. Occupational Therapy–trends. 3. Professional Role.
WM 450.5.O2 A244 2008]

RC487.A38 2008
616.89'165–dc22 2007019845
          MAC
A catalogue record for this title is available from the British Library

Set in Palatino 10/12.5
by Newgen Imaging Pvt Ltd, Chennai, India
Printed and bound in Singapore
by Fabulous Printers Pte Ltd

The publisher's policy is to use permanent paper from mills that operate a sustainable forestry policy,
and which has been manufactured from pulp processed using acid-free and elementary chlorine-free
practices. Furthermore, the publisher ensures that the text paper and cover board used have met
acceptable environmental accreditation standards.

For further information on Blackwell Publishing, visit our website:
www.blackwellpublishing.com

Contents

Contributors

Wendy Bryant MSc
School of Health Sciences and
   Social Care
Brunel University
Uxbridge, Middlesex
UK

Christine Craik MPhil
School of Health Sciences and
   Social Care
Brunel University
Uxbridge, Middlesex
UK

Samantha Dewis MSc
Penn Hospital
Wolverhampton
West Midlands, UK

Dr Carolyn Doughty
Balance NZ – Bipolar and Depression
   Network
Christchurch
New Zealand

Dr Edward A.S. Duncan
Nursing, Midwifery and Allied Health
   Professions Research Unit
University of Stirling
Stirling, Scotland
UK

Jacqueline Ede MSc
North East London Mental Health
   NHS Trust
Goodmayes Hospital
Ilford
Essex, UK

Michelle Harrison MA
Hallam Street Hospital
West Bromwich
West Midlands
UK

Elaine Hunter MSc
Royal Edinburgh Hospital
Morningside
Edinburgh, UK

Kee Hean Lim MSc
School of Health Sciences and
   Social Care
Brunel University
Uxbridge, Middlesex
UK

Dr Elizabeth Anne McKay
Department of Occupational
   Therapy
University of Limerick
Ireland

Karen L. Rebeiro Gruhl MSc
Sudbury Regional Hospital
Sudbury, Ontario
Canada

Gabrielle Richards MSc
South London & Maudsley
 NHS Foundation Trust
London
UK

Graeme Smith MA
Northumberland Tyne and
 Wear NHS Trust
Cherry Knowle Hospital
Sunderland, UK

Dr Thelma Sumsion
School of Occupational Therapy
Elborn College
University of Western Ontario
London, Ontario, Canada

Dr Samson Tse
Faculty of Medical and Health Sciences
University of Auckland
Auckland, New Zealand

Carla van Heerden
Employment and Vocational
 Opportunities
Mascalls Park Hospital
Brentwood, UK

Preface

Advancing practice in complex environs: mental health

Progress lies not in enhancing what is but in advancing towards what will be   (Kahill Gibran)

Occupational therapy evolved as a health and social care profession from the roots of psychiatry. Occupational therapists have worked with people with mental illness for over a century. It is accepted that psychiatry has changed and has been redefined since that time and that the emphasis for intervention has moved beyond the asylum of old to the multi-cultural community of today. Occupational therapy's contribution to mental health services internationally is significant, if under-recognised. That said, recent research from around the world demonstrates the importance of meaningful occupation to improve clients' health, their functioning and participation in their local neighbourhood.

The editors represent both practice and education, and all believe that occupational therapy has made, and should continue to make, that significant contribution to mental health practice. The editors include British, Australian and Singaporean therapists; the idea for this book grew from the belief that mental health continues to be a practice area within ever-changing contexts and dynamics and with particular challenges, and that expert narratives, whether from practitioners or researchers, are not well represented in the professional literature. Their stories of delivering or researching services in complex systems can offer real-world perspectives and useful insights to others.

Whiteford and Wright-St Clair (2005) highlight that complexity both challenges and explains our modern society, existing as it does at many levels. They define complexity as 'the richness and variety of structure and behaviour that arises from the interactions between the components of a system' (p. 5). It is the array of interactions and interconnections that make the health care and social systems in which we work complex environs. Rarely are occupational therapists required to find a simple solution to a client's problem – most often clients' problems are situated in contexts that demand intricate responses from practitioners.

Cowan (2006) discusses complexity in relation to higher education; here his perspective is related to occupational therapy. If we consider therapy as an outcome of an interaction between individuals and environments, and if we further consider that both therapist and client are interactions of their history, culture, thinking and emotions, then it follows that the result will be unpredictable, with interventions having unexpected outcomes. Given this, nothing in practice is certain and there is no correct answer; then, therapists must act well, in light of their understanding, experiences and research. This is advanced practice in action.

Professional practice knowledge refers to the knowledge base used by an individual or a profession including knowledge derived from theory, research and professional experience. Advanced practitioners develop practice wisdom. That is to say, practice wisdom generated from their *practice experience, cognitive* and *meta-cognitive processes* are linked in clinical reasoning, with professional judgements and the affective processes that together produce cultural competence (Higgs & Jones, 2000). These aspects form the basis of applying advanced professional knowledge in practice. To summarise, to become advanced practitioners, therapists must move beyond competent practice. They are required to be reflective, curious and creative: developing expertness in their own specific domain as well as being able to conduct and contribute to research and to educate others.

The need for advanced practitioners to deal with the ever-changing, complex, health and social care contexts worldwide is gaining in recognition. Fraser and Greenhaugh suggested that 'successful health services in the 21st century must aim not merely for change, improvement and response but for change-ability, improvability and responsiveness' (2001, p. 799). Advanced practitioners are seen as crucial elements to develop the health workforce and to modernise services. Esdaile and Ryan (2003).

> *outlined key elements of advanced practice. These included; breadth and depth of individual knowledge, appreciation of the wider context, critical thinking, continual striving to further develop knowledge and skills, often leading to additional qualifications and a commitment to quality. Typically such individuals also make a contribution to one or more areas of practice.* (p. 32)

The advanced practitioner is defined as being specialised or having highly developed knowledge and skills beyond those, which are required for registration, encompassing the breadth and depth of current and future professional practice (DOH, 2000).

This book captures and reflects current advanced occupational therapy practice, nationally and internationally. It showcases the innovative practice and research taking place in occupational therapy within mental health contexts. Throughout the text there is on emphasis on occupational therapists being specialists in occupation and for them to be specialists rather than generalists in the mental health arena. The authors articulate their expert knowledge and skills in their practice or research.

Finally, we hope that you are stimulated by the text that it speaks to you on many levels allowing you to reflect on your own practice and to consider how you can contribute to advancing occupational therapy in mental health in the future.

Elizabeth Anne McKay
Christine Craik
Kee Hean Lim
Gabrielle Richards

References

Brown G, Esdaile SA, Ryan SE (2003) *Becoming an Advanced Healthcare Practitioner*. Edinburgh: Butterworth Heinemann.

Cowan J (2006) *On Becoming an Innovative University Teacher: Reflection in Action*. Berkshire: Society for research into higher education and Open University Press.

Department of Health (DOH) (2000) *The NHS Plan*. London: HMSO.

Fraser SW, Greenhaugh T (2001) Coping with complexity: educating for capability. *British Medical Journal, 323(6 October)*, 799–803.

Higgs J, Jones M (2000) *Clinical Reasoning in the Health Professions*. Oxford: Butterworth Heinemann.

Whiteford G, Wright-St Clair, V (2005) *Occupation and Practice in Context*. Sydney: Elsevier Churchill Livingstone.

Part I Introducing the Mental Health Context

1 What have we been 'doing'?
A historical review of occupational therapy

Elizabeth Anne McKay

Personal narrative

Before I address the question of how occupational therapists got here, I will answer the question: how did I get here? What has influenced my knowledge and practice to bring me to my current work and research interests, and why this book?

I grew up in a working-class family living in a large Glasgow housing estate. My father worked and my mother kept the house. I was the eldest daughter with two older brothers and two younger sisters. It was an interesting position to inhabit. It was not until I was in my teens that my mother felt able to return to work. I am sure this was because I was now deemed able to take on board some of the household tasks that she left behind, for example, preparing evening meals. I believed at the time that my elder brothers were as capable as I was of cooking and serving up this meal but the task became mine. We were, after all, a traditional working-class household with easily identifiable women's tasks and men's jobs. It took me a while to realise things could be different.

I also grew up near one of Glasgow's largest mental hospitals. This meant that I had knowledge of psychiatry from a young age. At a superficial level, I was aware that the people that I often saw at my local shops looked different in their dress and general presentation. They were patients from the hospital. I had further opportunities to observe the inside of the mental hospital on my visits with local church groups to celebrate the main Christian festivities of Christmas and Easter. These visits were always interesting: I had a close-up view of the environment and of the patients, who seemed surprisingly ordinary. We were, of course, reminded on these occasions to be on our best behaviour. I later returned to this same hospital as I prepared for my interview at the Glasgow School of Occupational Therapy. On that occasion, I was allowed access to the patients within occupational therapy settings. Although my interest was stimulated, at this stage, I had decided my career in occupational therapy would be within physical settings. Perhaps, I was drawn to the uniform, its status and its power.

However, this decision changed on my first practice placement. I found myself, in 1983, in another mental hospital, this time in Dundee. This hospital upheld the Victorian ideal of asylum, being well away from the town; indeed, special transport arrangements existed to get staff to and from their place of work. I began to read about mental illness, not about the psychiatric conditions I witnessed but from a sociological perspective. I realised that psychiatry was an area that was little understood and that society preferred it to be out of sight. Nonetheless, during this placement, I was fortunate to be working in a setting that provided treatment to a range of patients who had acute and enduring mental health problems. I was fascinated by the lives of the people I met there. I was intrigued by the turns in their lives that had brought them into the psychiatric system. Some patients were on their first, frightening admission, and others had spent a lifetime (or so it seemed to me) in this hospital. I tried to understand the pressures and the inequalities that had resulted in people having mental illness.

It was against this background that I decided mental health would be my future area of practice. In my first post as an occupational therapist I worked in the long-stay wards of the Royal Edinburgh Hospital. Here were women who had been admitted to the psychiatric services for not adhering to society's norms of previous generations, for example, having an illegitimate child. The result was a lifetime spent in an institution. I often wondered about these women, their experiences and the child from whom they had been separated. Similarly, within acute wards, I found that women were often labelled manipulative or attention seeking, and that their role as main carers of children and others was hardly considered. The focus was on stabilising the woman's mental status and on discharging her back to her community, with little or no follow-up. The development of my interest in women with enduring mental illness grew from these experiences. How was it that women found themselves in these situations? How did the profession in which I worked, which was and continues to be largely dominated by women, contribute to the maintenance of the system?

It was not until I began to study women with enduring mental illness for my doctoral thesis, to read of women's own experiences and to explore women writing about women that I became interested in the women's movement and feminism. I came to this body of literature rather late in the day: it certainly was not part of my occupational therapy education, nor had it been an aspect of my other education. This literature helped me to reconsider and gain understanding of my own experiences and to further consider the role of women in society and, specifically, the inequalities and oppression experienced by women with mental illness. This summary, I hope, makes the influences on my life, practice and research more transparent.

Occupational therapy development

Returning to the question, how did occupational therapists get here? As we settle into the new century, it is perhaps timely to review occupational therapy over the past century. This chapter will consider the growth of occupational therapy and its unique relationship with the early development of psychiatry. It will briefly examine the parallel historical development of psychiatry and occupational therapy. It will also demonstrate that occupational therapy's development in the UK was, and still is, significantly influenced by American and Canadian perspectives on contemporary occupational therapy theory and research. The chapter will conclude with consideration of the influences impacting on mental health practice internationally.

In the UK, from medieval times until the eighteenth century, mentally ill people relied on the charity of the church for care. In the eighteenth century, the affluent mentally ill could be looked after in a variety of ways, 'in the homes of physicians or clergymen, or they could be confined to private madhouses' (Hume & Pullen, 1986, p. 3). However, for the poor, these choices were not available. It was not until the latter half of the eighteenth century and throughout the nineteenth century that changes began to take place in the psychiatric field.

At this time, Busfield asserts that 'value was placed on reason, and unreason in all its forms – madness, crime and poverty was banished in a great confinement' (1996, p. 70). As a result, from the 1760s onwards institutions such as workhouses, prisons and hospitals were purpose-built, but few hospitals were opened for the mentally ill. The eventual overcrowding and abuse of these individuals led to the first legislation for the mentally ill in 1774 (Hume & Pullen, 1986). The mad, it was felt, needed to be cared for in special places. The result was the creation of the asylums: these buildings, often located in rural settings, were to be the mainstay for managing the mentally ill for over a century. This legislation introduced 'certification, no person could be detained without the signature of a physician, a surgeon or an apothecary' (Hume & Pullen, 1986, p. 5). In the field of mental illness, this resulted in the power of the medical profession, at this time, a male domain, being enshrined in law.

The impact of moral treatment

The emerging philosophy of this time drew on the humanistic principles of the age of enlightenment that proposed that 'all men were made equal and governed by universal laws' (Kielhofner, 1983, p. 11). There was an emphasis on the humanity of individuals and the importance of the arts to humanity. Moral treatment, as an approach to the mentally ill, led Philippe Pinel to introduce work to the Bicetre Asylum for the Insane, Paris. He further prescribed physical activity and manual work, with the aim of reducing the use of external physical coercion. This regime led to the freeing of inmates from their restraints in 1793. His reforms were widely recognised and followed across Europe and North America (Paterson, 1997).

In the UK, William and Samuel Tuke, Quakers, founded and developed the York Retreat, a private hospital based on moral treatment. They believed that by treating patients as rational individuals, they could be re-educated. Re-education was hoped for by structuring the environment physically, socially and temporally. Engagement in normal daily activities, work-related activities and play created a total daily programme of organised occupations that minimised the disorganised behaviour of the mentally ill. Occupation as therapy was created – the forerunner of occupational therapy (Wilcock, 2001).

Although, Pinel and the Tukes are held in esteem as the liberators of the mentally ill, there are some dissenters, notably Foucault (1967), the French philosopher, who argued that the constraints of the new moral treatment were just as tight as the chains that had held the people before.

Nonetheless, there was a growing emphasis in the nineteenth century on the use of occupations concentrated within the mental health field (Paterson, 1997). Early examples exist from a variety of locations in the UK. In Scotland, at the Montrose Asylum and later at the Crichton Institution, Dr W. A. F. Browne was the 'foremost of the moral psychiatrists in Scotland' (Paterson, 1997, p. 181). He understood the role of motivation in the therapeutic use of occupation. Moral treatment was seen to be a success – if only in a few locations. As Corrigan (2001, p. 203) highlighted, 'moral treatment was unable to challenge its appropriation of the governance of the insane'.

The early proponents of moral treatment in the USA were also psychiatrists. They included Rush, Dutton and Meyer, all of whom played a major role in the formation of the profession of occupational therapy (Hopkins & Smith, 1993). Benjamin Rush, considered to be the father of American psychiatry, was the first to use the concepts of moral treatment and occupation. He, like the Tukes, was a Quaker. Towards the end of the nineteenth century, Meyer reiterated the importance of occupation and treatment. His work has had a significant impact on the development of the philosophy of occupational therapy in the USA (Meyer, 1997). It was Meyer who employed Eleanor Clarke Slagle as the director of occupational therapy at his hospital. She set up the first professional school for occupational therapists in Chicago in 1915, and is acknowledged annually by the American Occupational Therapy Association (AOTA) in the keynote lecture named after her.

Rush's nephew, William Rush Dutton, another psychiatrist, also advocated the use of occupations. In 1911, he conducted a series of classes on the use of recreation and occupation for nurses at his hospital. In 1915, Dutton published the first complete text on occupational therapy. He later became editor of the *Archives of Occupational Therapy* which eventually became the *American Journal of Occupational Therapy* in 1947.

At the start of the twentieth century in the UK, asylum standards had fallen, as staff shortages and overcrowding grew and maltreatment existed. Moral treatment could not be sustained against this background, with the result that most asylums provided only custodial care (Paterson, 1997). Rollin (2003, p. 297) in his retrospective 'Psychiatry in Britain one hundred years ago' argues that the early reformers' dreams were shattered and that 'the idealised asylums had become grossly overcrowded, under valued and under funded'. He concludes that restraint in the form of strait jackets and padded cells continued well into the twentieth century. Nonetheless, work activities were still used with patients, but more for the maintenance of the institution rather than for the benefit of those who were mentally ill. Exploitation was rife. Nonetheless, some smaller institutions continued to provide treatment regimes that held true to the value of occupation both for the individual's own productivity and for their personal satisfaction (Jackson, 1993). What is clear is that the reforming moral psychiatrists shared with the new profession of occupational therapy a belief in the efficacy of meaningful occupation as useful treatment in psychiatry. However, other world events also influenced the development of the profession.

Twentieth-century developments

A significant factor in the development of occupational therapy was the First World War. This saw rehabilitation centres set up throughout the UK to treat both physically and mentally injured soldiers, through the use of occupation. Other factors and international influences were also impacting and shaping the mental health field in 1920s. A Royal Commission (1924–1926) recommended that a special officer be appointed to each psychiatric hospital to direct patients' activities. In 1925, the first trained occupational therapist, Margaret Fulton, was employed at the Royal Cornhill Hospital, Aberdeen, Scotland. She had been educated in Philadelphia, America.

Dr D. K. Henderson introduced occupation into Gartnavel Royal Mental Hospital. In 1924, he presented a paper on occupational therapy to a meeting of the Royal Medico-Psychological Society of Mental Science. Dr Elizabeth Casson, the first woman doctor to graduate from Bristol University, heard him speak. She specialised in psychiatry, and this meeting prompted her to visit the USA and to later introduce occupational therapy to her psychiatric nursing home, Dorset House. She later sponsored the education of Constance Tebbit also at the Philadelphia School of Occupational Therapy. Tebbit along with Casson in 1930 founded Dorset House, the first occupational therapy school in the UK (Creek, 1990, p. 10). Elizabeth Casson today still influences contemporary occupational therapy through the provision of her trust fund, which supports education for occupational therapists and the Casson Memorial Lecture, which is the keynote address of the College of Occupational Therapists' annual conference.

In Scotland, the first school at the Astley Ainslie Hospital in Edinburgh was staffed by Canadian occupational therapists. In 1932, a group of 11 Scottish occupational therapists, mostly from psychiatric hospitals, formed the Scottish Association of Occupational Therapists. This became the first professional association in the UK. The influence of moral treatment, the growth of psychiatry as a medical specialism and both American and Canadian involvement have all influenced occupational therapy, and these aspects cannot be understated when reviewing the profession's development in the UK (Schemm, 1993).

External influences

There are many milestones in the development of psychiatric care in the UK from the 1930s onwards, including legislation, the founding of the National Health Service (NHS – 1948), the development of new drug treatments, especially major tranquillisers, and the move towards community care (Paterson, 1998). The work of Barton (1959) and Goffman (1961) highlighted the dehumanising ways in which patients were often treated in institutions, resulting in dependent and passive individuals. This added considerable weight to the demand for community-based services.

Mental health legislation and policy documents, for example, the Mental Treatment Act (1930), Hospital Services for the Mentally Ill (1971), the Mental Health Act (1983) and Caring for People (1989), show how consecutive governments aimed to improve mental health services. Most recently, governments have reinforced the refocusing of care to the community. The NHS Plan (Department of Health, 2000), the National Service Framework (NSF) for Mental Health (Department of Health, 1999) and the Scottish equivalent, the Framework for Mental Health Services (The Scottish Office, 1997), all advocate the further development of community care. Integration of health and social care agencies to provide effective care for people with enduring mental illness is embedded in these policies. Feaver (2000) stressed that to meet the aims of the NSF there must be a drive towards collaborative, continued professional development. These developments in the UK are mirrored in other countries.

The combined effects of these external factors have had a lasting impact on the shape of occupational therapy. The closure of large mental hospitals and the consequent reduction in bed numbers have resulted in many individuals with enduring mental health problems living in the community. Occupational therapists continue to work with individuals with a range of mental health problems, in many contexts. Some therapists still work in in-patient areas, some bridge the gap between hospital and community and others work solely in the community. Some are employed by the NHS, others by the Social Services and still others by non-statutory organisations. A growth area within mental health services has been the development of forensic occupational therapy services within the specialist State Mental Hospitals (Duncan *et al.*, 2003).

Internal influences

Internal pressures within the profession have also contributed to changing practice. The 1960s and 1970s saw the influence of a range of theories impacting occupational therapy in mental health, including analytical psychotherapy, behaviourism and cognitive theories (Kielhofner, 1983). The profession was in a time of crisis. The integration of such theories led to the loss of professional confidence and commitment to occupation. Reitz (1992) found that occupational therapy abandoned its earlier philosophy of occupation and health. Therapists had lost their appreciation of the importance of occupation and its significance to human life (Kielhofner, 1983; Whiteford, 2000).

These pressures were experienced not only in the UK but also in North America and Australia. The profession identified a growing need among therapists for a unifying concept. In the 1980s, the refocus on humans as occupational beings with occupation and occupational performance being identified as core concepts of the profession led to the development of practice models: for example, Reed and Sanderson (1980), Model of Human Occupation (Kielhofner, 1985) and The Canadian

Model of Occupational Performance (CAOT, 1997). These models have strengthened therapists' belief in their profession and in the health-giving benefits of the occupation. They have enabled most therapists to articulate the complexity of occupational therapy and the significance of the person–environment–occupation relationship.

Within the UK, occupational therapy in mental health is still a significant area of practice, with approximately one-third of therapists being employed (Walker & Lynham, 1999). However, this is not the case in other Western countries. In the recent Canadian Association of Occupational Therapists Membership Statistics (CAOT, 2005) 12.3 % of occupational therapists reported their main practice setting as mental health. In a recent workforce survey by AOTA of 8998 occupational therapists and occupational therapy assistants; 3195 responded. Of these respondents, 3.6% indicated that their primary work setting was in mental health and a further 3.5% indicated that their secondary work setting was mental health. (personal communication, AOTA, 2006). Australia traditionally had fewer therapists employed in mental health practice; recent figures from the OT Australia indicate that, of their total membership of 4592, only 602 (15%) therapists are listed as working in mental health (personal communication, OT Australia, 2006). Ireland, too, has traditionally had a smaller number of occupational therapists working in the mental health arena; the Association of Occupational Therapists Ireland (personal communication, AOTI) indicates that approximately 120 therapists (10%) work in mental health settings in Ireland.

Given that occupational therapy has its roots in mental health, the small proportion of therapists working in this area has been a matter of concern. There is an ongoing debate about the specific contribution of occupational therapy in mental health. In an attempt to address these issues, in the 1990s, the College of Occupational Therapists, in the UK, established a Mental Health Project Working Group to produce a position paper on the way ahead for research, education and practice in mental health. It identified little research literature relating to the practice and management of occupational therapy in mental health (Craik, 1998; Craik et al., 1999). As a result, two surveys were undertaken to profile practitioners and managers working in mental health.

The first survey, by Craik et al. (1998), explored the views of practitioners. This work identified that issues existed around role definition, the need for a unifying theory and research, and the value of the profession. Nevertheless, the respondents were committed and enthusiastic about occupational therapy in mental health. Although few of the respondents had direct involvement in research, most were aware of the need for research and evidence-based practice.

The second survey examined the perspectives of occupational therapy managers in mental health. It revealed that the majority of mangers were women. In the main, similar findings to the practitioners' survey were found. These findings included the need for clarification of the core skills, roles and approaches of occupational therapists (Craik et al., 1999).

Building on the work by Craik et al. (1999), Fowler-Davis and Bannigan (2000) explored the priorities for mental health research in the UK. They identified the three areas most needing research to be occupation, group work and occupational performance skills. They further identified that the core skills of the profession, professional status, effectiveness issues and finally, client-centredness, were all worthy of further research. An update of the mental health research priorities by Fowler-Davis and Hyde (2002) indicated that occupation remained the number-one research priority area; however, occupational performance and users' perspectives were ranked second (3 in 1999) and third (8 in 1999). respectively. The position of users' perspective marked the greatest change from the 1999 priorities, reflecting the need to involve service users in research, service design and provision. The message of these surveys was clear: occupational therapists were questioning their unique contribution and their status within mental health services.

Duncan (1999) emphasises that one way to silence the continued call for clarification of the profession's contribution is evidence-based research into the efficacy of occupational therapy and occupation. Wilcock (1999) takes this further advocating for research and intervention at policy and population levels focusing on enabling occupation, health and well-being. Whatever form the research takes, it requires involving service users in its development, implementation and evaluation. Only such collaborative research can create a firm evidence base for occupational therapy to provide effective services to its users in both health and social care settings.

Building the evidence base

Recently, there has been some movement towards bridging the research gap in UK mental health practice. Studies conducted across a range of topics include:

- The role of primary mental health care in meeting the needs of people with enduring mental health problems (Cook, 1997; Cook & Howe, 2003).
- The quality-of-life priorities for people with enduring mental health problems (Mayers, 2000).
- Support groups for people who have experienced psychosis (Hyde, 2001).
- Clinical effectiveness and the Canadian Occupational Performance Measure (Chesworth et al., 2002).

Significantly, over the last decade, occupational science has developed as an academic discipline to generate knowledge about the form, function and meaning of human occupation (Zemke & Clarke, 1996). Occupational science is a multi-professional discipline, initially developed at the University of Southern California. It built on the work of Meyer, Riley, Ayres and others, and the ideas put forward have generated worldwide interest and research (Yerxa et al., 1989). It is argued that occupational therapy's unique contribution to health lies in the relationship between health and occupation (Wilcock, 1998). Wilcock and others have argued that there is a human biological need for occupation (Wilcock, 1993; Wood, 1998)

Wilcock (1998) stressed that occupational therapy has latterly concentrated on ill health and that the profession has negated the potential of occupation to influence the public health agenda. She has worked to explore this perspective and, in the process, has repositioned occupational therapy beyond its traditional health and social care borders. Occupational science as a theory has offered occupational therapists' new ways of thinking and new ideas to broaden the profession's horizon (Wilcock, 2001).

Occupational science proposes that individuals should be studied in their interactions with their occupations and environment in everyday situations (Yerxa *et al.*, 1989). It draws upon a multi-professional background and recognises the need for a variety of research methods that enable the illumination of our understanding of how people ascribe meaning to occupation and their lives. Methods to achieve these aims have focused on using qualitative methods, including narrative inquiry, to access and present diverse accounts (Polkinghorne, 1995; Frank, 1996). These methods are consistent with the central tenets of post-modernism, with its emphasis on different perspectives, situatedness, temporality and contexts. Occupational science has unified a focus on occupation and facilitated alternative research to be undertaken.

In a review of 6 years of *British Journal of Occupational Therapy* from January 2000 to September 2006, the influence of occupational science is readily evident. There has been an increase in mental-health-related publications with authors responding to the call for research involving users of mental health services to explore occupation and the relationship between health, well-being and engagement in occupation. Time-use (Shimitras *et al.*, 2003; Farnworth *et al.*, 2004; Bejerholm *et al.*, 2006), the value of occupation (Mee *et al.*, 2004), barriers to occupational engagement (Chugg & Craik, 2002) and the meanings engagement in occupation adds to their lives have all been researched. Furthermore, the occupations explored took place in a variety of contexts; in-patient and forensic units, day services and community settings. These studies encompass a range of occupations including adult education (Westwood, 2003), horticulture (Fieldhouse, 2003), leisure and outdoor recreation (Heasman & Atwal, 2004; Craik & Pieris, 2006; Frances, 2006), skills acquisition, life skills training (Mairs & Bradshaw, 2004), woodwork (Mee & Sumsion, 2001), cooking (Hayley & McKay, 2004) and support groups (Hyde, 2001).

These studies demonstrate the importance of occupation to the lives of people with mental health problems. Although all are based on relatively small samples, they contribute to a growing body of research that explores the perspectives of mental health users. They begin to address the significance of occupation to maintaining mental health and they further explore, in some depth, the meaning that individuals ascribe to their lives through occupation. The body of work makes a valuable contribution to evidence-based mental health practice, revealing the importance of positive and successful experiences through participating in occupations leading to a sense of meaning, increased self-esteem, skill acquisition and an improved sense of identity. The importance of supportive environments, opportunities for social networking, facilitating people to make their own choices and, importantly, enabling them to take control of their lives were to the fore.

The work to date goes some way to address the earlier calls for relevant research and it reflects the research priorities identified by Fowler-Davis and Bannigan (2000). This research offers a sound foundation on which the College of Occupational

Therapy can move forward with its 10-year Mental Health Strategy for Occupational Therapists (2006). The strategy highlights five key themes: occupation focused, person centred, accessible, available and relevant (COT, 2006).

Current influences on occupational therapists working in metal health

The international influences on therapists practising in mental health currently include the recovery movement, users' perspectives and participation, social inclusion, vocational rehabilitation and cultural sensitivity. Practice contexts that continue to challenge occupational therapists are acute care, crisis intervention and forensic settings. The chapters of this book follow a broadly similar format of a personal narrative through which the scene is set for the author's journey in mental health, exploration of the evidence for their practice and examples of advanced practice. However, contributors have adopted different approaches to fulfil their remit of writing a chapter, reflecting the diversity of mental health practice. Some have shared a very personal narrative that has influenced practice while others have shared their research or research careers. Each chapter concludes with a number of key questions to assist readers in thinking about the chapter content in relation to advancing their practice.

A brief glance at the list of authors and their current affiliation gives some indication of their international background, but closer examination reveals even more diverse experience. Authors currently work in occupational therapy in practice, education and research in the UK, Ireland, Canada and New Zealand. But if their country of origin is noted, other countries are represented: South Africa, Singapore, Australia and Hong Kong. Several authors received their occupational therapy education and practised in one country before moving to another; so, Carla van Heerden from South Africa is now practising in London; Kee Hean Lim from Singapore is now teaching in London and Samson Tse from Hong Kong is now living and researching in New Zealand as is Caroline Doughty. Thelma Sumsion was educated in Canada and practised and taught there before moving to England, where she taught and undertook her PhD in London before returning to Canada. The authors represent a truly international perspective on the current influences and practice.

Anthony (2000) considers that 'recovery is a process...a belief which infuses a system...which providers can hold for service users...grounded on the idea that people can recover form mental illness and that the delivery system must be constructed on this knowledge' (p. 159). Recovery highlights practice based on restoring hope, making meaning, experiencing success, taking control and maintaining and developing supportive relationships (Repper & Perkins, 2003). In the last 15 years there has been an increased interest in incorporating recovery philosophy into services particularly in New Zealand, Canada, the US, the UK and Ireland. Recovery and occupational therapy are considered in depth by Karen Rebeiro in Chapter 8.

Social inclusion and its relationship to mental health problems is well recognised and complex. Users of mental health services can be excluded in multiple ways and experience stigma and discrimination in their daily lives. Occupational engagement and community participation are highlighted as ways of reducing both stigma and discrimination. Wendy Bryant offers a stimulating discussion on occupational alienation and inclusion within the community in Chapter 7.

The importance of work to increase engagement and social inclusion is discussed by Carla van Heerdan in Chapter 10 as she merges her South African and UK experiences of vocational rehabilitation. The use of creative activities in community settings offers a possible way forward to enhance social inclusion and reduce alienation in the community. In Chapter 9, Jacqueline Ede illustrates innovative partnerships to achieve inclusion.

In Chapter 2 Gabrielle Richards provides an overview of the impact of policy on occupational therapy practice. Cultural sensitivity and multiculturalism pose challenges for services worldwide, and in Chapter 3, Kee Hean Lim reviews the significance of cultural sensitivity in practice.

In Chapters 4 and 5, Samantha Dewis and Michelle Harrison discuss the importance of occupational therapy in acute care and crisis intervention teams. Elaine Hunter shares her experiences of developing a forensic service aligned to the best evidence in Chapter 6. Graeme Smith in Chapter 11 reinforces the significance of narrative to change the dominant discourses prevalent in mental health.

The need for users to be active participants, collaborators and consultants in service provision, development and research is well established. In Chapter 12, Dr Samson Tse and Dr Carolyn Doughty present the results of a systematic review examining user participation in service delivery. In Chapters 13 and 14 Dr Edward Duncan and Dr Thelma Sumsion, respectively, share their personal journeys as researchers. To conclude, in Chapter 15 Christine Craik reflects on the past and offer insights into possible futures for occupational therapy in mental health.

Questioning your practice

1. Reflect on your career to date how you have got to where you are?
2. How has your practice changed in the past 2 years?
3. How do you imagine your future practice developing?

References

American Association of Occupational Therapists (2006) Personal communication.

Anthony WA (2000) A recovery-oriented service system. Setting some system standards. *Psychiatric Réhabilitation Journal, 24(2)*, 159–168.

Barton R (1959) *Institutional Neurosis*. Bristol: Wright.

Bejerholm U, Hansson L, Eklund M (2006) Profiles of occupational engagement in people with schizophrenia (POES): The development of a new instrument based on time use diaries. *British Journal of Occupational Therapy, 6(2)*, 58–68.

Busfield J (1996) *Men, Women and Madness: Understanding Gender and Mental Disorder.* London: Macmillan Press.

Canadian Association of Occupational Therapy (CAOT) (1997) *Enabling Occupation: An Occupational Therapy Perspective.* Ottawa: Canadian Association of Occupational Therapy.

CAOT (2005) *Canadian Association of Occupational Therapists Membership Statistics.* Ottawa: Canadian Association of Occupational Therapy.

Chesworth C, Duffy R, Hodnett J, Knight A (2002). Measuring clinical effectiveness in mental health: Is the Canadian Occupational Performance an appropriate measure? *British Journal of Occupational Therapy, 65(1),* 31–34.

Chugg A, Craik C (2002) Some factors influencing occupational engagement for people with schizophrenia living in the community. *British Journal of Occupational Therapy, 65(2),* 67–74.

College of Occupational Therapy (2006) *Recovery Ordinary Lives: The Strategy for Occupational Therapy in Mental Health Services 2007–2017.* London: COT.

Cook S (1997) *Results of the Needs Assessment Survey 1996 and Proposals for Service Development.* Sheffield: Pitsmoor Surgery.

Cook, S, Howe A (2003) Engaging people with enduring psychotic conditions in primary mental health care and occupational therapy. *British Journal of Occupational Therapy, 66(6),* 236–246.

Corrigan K (2001) Doing time in mental health: Discipline at the edge of medicine. *British Journal of Occupational Therapy, 64(4),* 203–205.

Craik C (1998) Occupational therapy in mental health: a review of the literature. *British Journal of Occupational Therapy, 61(5),* 186–192.

Craik C, Chacksfield JD, Richards, G (1998) A survey of occupational therapy practitioners in mental health. *British Journal of Occupational Therapy, 61(5),* 227–234.

Craik C, Austin C, Schell D (1999) A national survey of occupational therapy managers in mental health. *British Journal of Occupational Therapy, 62(5),* 220–228.

Craik C, Pieris Y (2006) Without leisure… 'It wouldn't be much of a life': the meaning of leisure for people with mental health problems. *British Journal of Occupational Therapy, 69(5),* 209–216.

Creek J (Ed.) (1990) *Occupational Therapy and Mental Health: Principles, Skills and Practice.* Edinburgh: Churchill Livingstone.

Department of Health (1983) *The Mental Health Act.* London: HMSO.

Department of Health (1999) *National Service Framework for Mental Health: Modern Standards and Service Models.* London: HMSO.

Department of Health (2000) *The NHS Plan.* London: HMSO.

Duncan E (1999) Occupational therapy in mental health: It is time to recognise that it has come of age? *British Journal of Occupational Therapy, 62(11),* 521–522.

Duncan E, Munro K, Nicol M (2003) Research priorities in forensic occupational therapy. *British Journal of Occupational Therapy, 62(2),* 55–64.

Farnworth L, Nikitin L, Fossey E (2004) Being in a secure forensic psychiatric unit: Every day is the same, killing time or making the most of it. *British Journal of Occupational Therapy, 67(10),* 430–438.

Feaver S (2000) The new policy for mental health services. *British Journal of Occupational Therapy, 63(4),* 147.

Fieldhouse J (2003) The impact of an allotment group on mental health clients' health, wellbeing and social networking. *British Journal of Occupational Therapy (66)7,* 286–296.

Foucault M (1967). *Madness and Civilisation: A History of Insanity in the Age of Reason.* London: Tavistock.

Fowler-Davis S, Bannigan K (2000) Priorities in mental health research: The results of a live research project. *British Journal of Occupational Therapy, 63(3)*, 98–104.

Fowler-Davis S, Hyde P (2002) Priorities in mental health research: An update. *British Journal of Occupational Therapy, 65(8)*, 387–389.

Frances K (2006) Outdoor recreation as an occupation to improve quality of life for people with enduring mental health problems. *British Journal of Occupational Therapy, 69(4)*, 182–186.

Frank G (1996) Life histories in occupational therapy clinical practice. *American Journal of Occupational Therapy, 50(4)*, 251–264.

Goffman E (1961) *Asylums*. Harmondsworth: Penguin.

Haley L, McKay EA (2004) 'Baking gives you confidence': Users' views of engaging in the occupation of baking. *British Journal of Occupational Therapy, 67(3)*, 125–128.

Heasman D, Atwal A (2004) The active advice pilot project: Leisure enhancement and social inclusion for people with severe mental health problems. *British Journal of Occupational Therapy, 67(11)*, 511–514.

Hopkins HL, Smith HD (1993) *Williard and Spackman's Occupational Therapy* (5th edn). Philadelphia, PA: Lippincott.

Hume C, Pullen I (1986) *Rehabilitation in Psychiatry*. Edinburgh: Churchill Livingstone.

Hyde P (2001) Support groups for people who have experienced psychosis. *British Journal of Occupational Therapy, 64(4)*, 169–174.

Jackson M (1993) From work to therapy: The changing politics of occupation in the twentieth century. *British Journal of Occupational Therapy, 56(10)*, 360–364.

Kielhofner G (1983) *Health through Occupation: Theory and Practice in Occupational Therapy*. Philadelphia, PA: F. A. Davis.

Kielhofner G (1985) *A Model of Human Occupation: Theory and Application*. Baltimore, MD: Williams & Wilkins.

Mayers CA (2000) Quality of life: Priorities for people with enduring mental health problems. *British Journal of Occupational Therapy, 63(12)*, 591–597.

Mairs H, Bradshaw T (2004) Life skills training in schizophrenia. *British Journal of Occupational Therapy, 67(5)*, 217–224.

Mee J, Sumsion T (2001) Mental health clients confirm the motivating power of occupation. *British Journal of Occupational Therapy, 64(3)*, 121–128.

Mee J, Sumsion T, Craik C (2004) Mental health clients confirm the value of occupation in building competence and self-identity. *British Journal of Occupational Therapy, 67(5)*, 225–233.

Meyer A (1997) The philosophy of occupational therapy. *American Journal of Occupational Therapy, (31)*, 639–642 (original article 1922).

Paterson CF (1997) Rationales for the use of occupation in 19th Century Asylums. *British Journal of Occupational Therapy, 60(4)*, 179–183.

Paterson CF (1998) Occupational therapy and the National Health Service, 1948–1998. *British Journal of Occupational Therapy, 61(7)*, 311–315.

Polkinghorne DE (1995) Narrative configuration in qualitative analysis. *Qualitative Studies in Education, 8(1)*, 5–23.

Reed K, Sanderson SR (1980) *Concepts of Occupational Therapy*. Baltimore, MD: Williams & Wilkins.

Reitz SM (1992) A historical review of occupational therapy's role in preventive health and wellness. *American Journal of Occupational Therapy, 46(1)*, 50–55.

Repper J, Perkins R (2003) *Social Inclusion and Recovery: A Model for Mental Health Practice*. Edinburgh: Baillière Tindall.

Rollins HR (2003) Psychiatry in Britain one hundred years ago. *British Journal of Psychiatry, (183)*, 292–298.

Schemm RL (1993) Bridging conflicting ideologies: The origins of American and British occupational therapy. *American Journal of Occupational Therapy, 48(11)*, 1082–1088.

Shimitras L, Fossey E, Harvey C (2003) Time use of people living with schizophrenia in North London. *British Journal of Occupational Therapy, 66(2)*, 46–54.

The Scottish Office (1997) *A Framework for Mental Health Services in Scotland*. Edinburgh: The Scottish Office.

Walker C, Lynham C (1999) *Numbers and Areas of Practice of Occupational Therapists Working in Mental Health Services in Great Britain*. Ripon and York: Department of Health.

Westwood J (2003) The impact of adult education for mental health service users. *British Journal of Occupational Therapy, 66(11)*, 505–510.

Whiteford G (2000) Occupational deprivation: Global challenge in the new millennium. *British Journal of Occupational Therapy, 63(5)*, 200–204.

Wilcock AA (1993) A theory of the human need for occupation. *Occupational Science, 1(1)*, 17–24.

Wilcock AA (1998) *An Occupational Perspective of Health*. Thorofare, NJ: Slack Incorporated.

Wilcock, AA (1999) The Doris Sym Memorial Lecture: Developing a philosophy of occupation for health. *British Journal of Occupational Therapy, 62(5)*, 192–198.

Wilcock AA (2001) Occupational science: The key to broadening horizons. *British Journal of Occupational Therapy, 64(8)*, 412–417.

Wood W (1998) Biological requirement for occupation in primates: An explanatory study and theoretical analysis. *Journal of Occupational Science, (5)*, 66–81.

Yerxa EJ, Clark F, Frank G, Jackson J, Parnham D, Pierce D, Stein C, Zemke R (1989) An introduction to occupational science: A foundation for occupational therapy in the 21st Century. *Occupational Therapy in Health Care, 6*, 1–17.

Zemke R, Clarke F (Eds) (1996) *Occupational Science: The Evolving Discipline*. Philadelphia, PA: F. A. Davis.

2 The changing face of occupational therapy in mental health

Gabrielle Richards

Personal narrative

I am the professional head of occupational therapy at the South London and Maudsley Foundation National Health Service (NHS) Trust, responsible for professional advice to the occupational therapy service and line management of physiotherapy and dietetic services. The Trust's mental health and substance misuse division provides services to a local population of over 1 million people across four London boroughs as well as specialist services for the UK. I am also the past chair of the College of Occupational Therapists Specialist Section in Mental Health (formally the Association of Occupational Therapists in Mental Health).

I had always known that I would work in mental health. It just felt right. As an occupational therapy student, my practice placements in mental health were the most rewarding and meaningful. Throughout my career in Australia and later in the UK, mental health has been my passion.

I have worked in various settings, starting in a rehabilitation service for older adults with severe and enduring mental health problems. Then travel intervened, and I worked as a locum occupational therapist, before moving to a community post that covered all aspects of care. One day I would take equipment to an older adult in the community, see someone with a mental health problem and, the next day, deliver an anxiety management course in the community and present a disability awareness workshop in the local primary school: an all-encompassing practice. After a short time in a lecturing post, I returned to mental health, and there I remained.

Being an occupational therapist in mental health has never disappointed me. Despite the frustrations of different work settings and practices and constant changes there is something quite comforting about knowing my profession has a significant role to play in enhancing the lives of people who experience mental health difficulties.

In preparing this chapter, I reflected on where I am today, my motivations and, in particular, my interest in policy and its influence over practice and the development of the profession. I have taken opportunities to engage with my profession and the wider context in which it operates. I believe whole heartedly in occupational therapists getting involved with their professional body and influencing the direction of the profession to secure our place in mental health provision.

Introduction

This chapter will look at the changing face of occupational therapy in mental health, bringing the story up to date and exploring the contexts and developments of occupational therapy within the UK. Although the changes relate principally to the UK, there are parallels in other countries.

I propose that occupational therapy's central tenet has not changed. Occupational therapy's uniqueness is its focus on occupation and the belief that it is vital to maintaining and promoting people's health and well-being (Creek, 2003; COT, 2006a). *The Strategy for Occupational Therapy for Mental Health* (COT, 2006a) suggests that occupational engagement is important to the thinking of occupational therapists. This leads to a focus on the strengths of individuals, rather than their problems, and contributes to their recovery journey. As Ormston (2006, p. 102) wrote 'whilst we might develop new ways to practice occupational therapy, and occupational therapists might take on wide-ranging roles, underlying principles and values remain constant'.

Forever changing are the contexts and the policy/political drives that affect the practice and environments in which the profession operates. Whilst occupational therapy continues to have a strong role in in-patient services, day services and community settings, the struggle is to ensure and maintain the unique contribution of the profession as services and philosophy change direction. It has been suggested that occupational therapy has been reactive to policy changes, but more recently there has been a significant shift to a more proactive stance to its mental health policy. (Craik *et al.*, 1998a; COT, 2006a)

There are developing influences within the UK that the profession needs to address and shape. These influences are not mutually exclusive but are interwoven: the political and policy landscape, mental health and social inclusion, workforce modernisation and new and extended roles and new ways of working. In discussing these influences, examples of occupational therapy involvement will be highlighted; although centred on the UK developments, they have international resonance.

The political and policy landscape

Mental health was identified as a key government priority for service improvement and modernisation in the National Service Framework (NSF) (DH, 1999). It set out the detailed direction and goals for improving mental health in England. It addressed the mental health needs of adults up to 65 years of age. It set national standards, service models and programmes to underpin the implementation of integrated local services. It also had a series of national milestones and performance indicators to ensure effective performance management. The standards related to mental health promotion, discrimination/exclusion, primary care, access to services, services for people with severe mental health problems, support for carers and action to reduce suicides. To support the implementation of the framework, there has been an unprecedented amount of policy, guidance and investment.

However, as Ormston (1999) reflected, although the document did not refer specifically to occupational therapy, the framework advocated a bio-psychosocial approach with emphasis on meeting service users' occupational, social, leisure needs and activities of daily living. In reality, the document had much to offer to occupational therapists and the direction they could take. Much of this is now in place – for example, the refocus on socially inclusive practice, new ways of working and extended roles for the professional and non-professional workforce.

McCulloch, Glover and St John (2003) suggested that the framework was far reaching and crucial in the development of modern mental health policy. Following the NSF, the National Health Service Plan (DH, 2000a) set specific targets for three new kinds of specialist teams: assertive outreach, crisis resolution/home treatment and early intervention in psychosis. These concentrated on intensive community care and much of the focus of funding was dominated by the implementation of these teams.

The presence of occupational therapists in these teams was initially limited, but since they became more established, occupational therapists are routinely found working in these teams either in an identified occupational therapy post or in a generic post. These different styles of working reflect the long-standing debate about occupational therapy specific versus generic working (Meeson, 1998a, 1998b; Craik *et al.*, 1998b). The College of Occupational Therapists advised that 'Occupational therapists should spend the majority of their clinical time working as occupational therapists and not as generalist mental health workers' (Craik *et al.*, 1998b, p. 391). However, there appears to be little evidence that this recommendation has been adopted by practitioners, and much of the literature continues to focus on the frustrations and dilemmas of generic versus specific occupational therapy practice. For example, Harries and Gilhooly (2003) reported that occupational therapists in community mental health teams have three ways of working: specifically as an occupational therapist, solely as a generic coordinator and a combination of these roles to varying degrees.

The 5-year review of the *NSF for Mental Health* (DH, 2004a) recommended some additional priorities: in-patient care, dual diagnoses, social exclusion; ethnic minorities, care of people with long-term mental disorders, availability of psychological therapies, better information and information systems, workforce redesign and new roles for key workers.

As the Sainsbury Centre for Mental Health (2005) reported mental health services in the UK have changed considerably over the past 20 years. With mental health being acknowledged to be a high-priority growth area, there has been a proliferation of activity around redesigning provision away from traditional services to more diverse service models. There has been a focus on increasing service user involvement, outreach day care, 24-h access, home-based support and evidence-based practice.

As the mental health agenda expanded, the College of Occupational Therapists recognised a need to consider the implications for practitioners. This also included a need for leadership and vision to promote the centrality of occupation to health and well-being and to address the policy drivers impacting on the delivery of services across the UK. This resulted in publication of the Strategy for Occupational Therapy in Mental Health Services (COT, 2006a).

Mental health and social inclusion

Although all the new priorities identified in the 5-year review of the *NSF for Mental Health* (DH, 2004a.) relate to occupational therapists, the social exclusion agenda is of paramount importance. The publication of the Mental Health and Social Exclusion Report (Office of the Deputy Prime Minister, 2004) gave a clear signal about the changes needed in mental health policy and practice in the UK. It outlined a plan to reduce and remove barriers to employment, to facilitate access to mainstream services and to encourage community participation for those with mental health problems. It also promoted government departments working together to support an integrated approach. It outlined seven project areas: employment, income and benefits, community participation, housing, education, direct payments and social networks.

Occupational therapists believe that the profession has always aimed to support people to be socially included, and therefore they welcomed the report that emphasised employment and vocational opportunities. However, in recent years the profession in the UK has neglected this important area and this report served as a potential vehicle to reinstate employment as a focus within practice. The College of Occupational Therapists (2006a) supports this development and predicts that more therapists will work in settings which emphasise employment and vocational opportunities as well as in potential areas, the report highlighted, in relation to reducing stigma and discrimination and promoting positive mental health and individual's social participation. Earlier, Robdale (2004) had commented that the profession needs to grab this opportunity to re-involve itself in this core area of practice and to develop vocational specialists.

The government, being committed to reducing the number of people with mental health problems on Incapacity Benefits (Department for Work and Pensions, 2006), is encouraging mental health services to support people with severe and enduring mental health problems to access vocational and employment opportunities (DH, 2006). Consequently, there are many opportunities and settings in which occupational therapy expertise could be, and is being, utilised.

Related to this, a number of occupational therapists are engaged in the national pilot 'Pathways to Work' projects around the country, where they are employed to promote and develop 'early return to work' programmes that give ongoing support to both the employee and to the employer.

Occupational therapists are now increasingly involved in the Condition Management Programme (CMP), a new initiative delivered in partnership with the NHS, designed to help people understand and manage their health condition in a work environment. The College of Occupational Therapists (2006b) has highlighted that occupational therapists are well placed to provide services to work environments to initiate and develop strategies to promote employee and organisational health using a range of client-centred, holistic occupational interventions within condition management.

Another issue gaining momentum is recovery. As the National Institute for Mental Health England (NIMHE, 2005) reported that recovery is a concept that was primarily introduced by people who had recovered from mental health experiences. They acknowledged that recovery has many different meanings within mental health and substance misuse services; primarily, it is not what services do to people but what individuals experience as they become empowered to achieve a fulfilling and meaningful life. For occupational therapists this may appear to be familiar territory. For example, NIMHE (2005) highlights the domains for recovery as: child care, family support, peer support and relationships, work/meaningful activity, power and control, stigma, community involvement, access to resources and education. These domains are congruent with those of occupational therapy as illustrated by Creek (2003) and Rebeiro Gruhl (2005).

But it is not enough to accept the similarities; occupational therapists must critique their practice in light of new concepts such as the recovery movement. The recovery model might be a paradigm shift for some professions: for occupational therapy it is an opportunity for the profession's long-held values of empowerment of the individual to be acknowledged and to facilitate more collaborative working with our multi-disciplinary colleagues. Allott *et al.* (2002) suggest that, if we adopt recovery in the UK, it will lead to new ways of working that challenge professional coercion. It is equally dependent on a radical shift in perceptions of what mental illness is and the maturing of methods of conceiving, approaching and treating it. Therefore, the plethora of new ways of working, new teams and government policy that put users at the centre of services are already integral to the ethos of occupational therapy.

Workforce modernisation

There has been much emphasis on the need to modernise education and training if the NHS workforce is to be equipped to deliver mental health services in the future. The Sainsbury Centre for Mental Health (1997) highlighted the need to ensure that the skills, knowledge and attitudes of both existing and future mental health staff are appropriate to the demands of the changing environments and evolving services. In this report, occupational therapy was identified as providing, possibly, the best model for professional input to community mental health teams.

Here, too there has been much guidance on new roles and new ways of working in mental health. Examples of this include Community Development Workers for the Black and Minority Ethnic Community (DH, 2004b), Support Time and Recovery Workers (DH, 2003a) and Graduate Workers for Primary Care (DH, 2003b).

The National Workforce Programme (NIMHE, 2004a), a part of the Care Services Improvement Partnership published a National Mental Health Workforce Strategy.

It aimed to improve workforce design, local planning and delivery; to identify and use creative means for recruitment and retention; to facilitate new ways of working across professional boundaries; to create new roles to attract new employees to complement existing staff; to develop the workforce through revised education and training at both pre- and post-qualification levels and, finally, to develop leadership and change management skills.

As, this workforce redesign also supports the development of a competency-based rather than a professionally educated workforce, occupational therapists need to ensure their place within it. For example, *The Ten Essential Shared Capabilities* (NIMHE, 2004b) advocated for staff working with people with mental health problems were developed following user and carer consultation. These capabilities were to be applicable to all staff groups regardless of qualification, and they were viewed as fundamental building blocks across health, social care and the non-statutory sectors.

New roles and extended roles

Linked to modernising the workforce, are the extended roles and new roles for staff in mental health services. The impetus for extended scope practice came from the increasing pressures and demands placed on health and social care services such as increased waiting lists, the need to improve continuity and quality of care and shortage of staff. The need has led to a re-examination of existing staffing structures and boundaries as defined in the Extended Scope of Practice Briefing (COT, 2006c). These imply working outside or beyond the recognised elements of occupational therapy, using skills and techniques that are not included in the defined core skills of an occupational therapist and/or are not included in the pre-registration education curriculum.

This is particularly relevant to mental health, where it has long been reported that there will be an insufficient staff to meet the requirements of a more flexible and diverse workforce. As the Kings Fund (2006) highlights, alternative approaches are needed to develop a responsive and sustainable workforce able to manage the complex changes and pressures facing the NHS. The report emphasises smarter working is needed rather than increasing the number of people employed. It challenges the professions to think and work differently and adopt new practices.

This perceived resistance to change may relate less to occupational therapy than other professions. As discussed earlier, occupational therapy's struggle is to ensure that the focus of valuing occupation for individuals is retained within current posts and new ways of working rather than resisting change. There are many examples of innovation in occupational therapy, and Pathways to Work and Condition Management Programmes are good examples as highlighted previously.

The College of Occupational Therapists (2003), for example, issued guidance on the workforce initiative of Support Time and Recovery (STR) Workers. Although their role could be viewed as similar to that of occupational therapy support workers, the College published measured guidance informing the profession about them and how occupational therapists could work with them. This mature and helpful approach was driven by service user needs and not professional ones. STR workers are a reality and many organisations and occupational therapists are now supporting and championing their development.

For example, within the South London and Maudsley Foundation Trust, the work to develop the STR worker role in one borough was taken forward by the head occupational therapist for Community Services and the Service Manager.

It started with a service review that resulted in the closure of day care services. Four posts, three occupational therapy technical instructors and one nursing assistant, were re-deployed to community mental health teams, and it seemed prudent to use the opportunity to undertake some review of these roles to promote these posts as STR workers. But work needed to be done to examine how current post holders were working in terms of adherence to the concept of STR workers.

A borough-wide audit was conducted to record the numbers and location of potential STR workers in other parts of the service. These have now increased to six STR workers, one in each of the four community mental health teams, one in the forensic community team and one in the assertive outreach teams.

It is important to recognise that the head occupational therapist had been involved in the auditing process, led on the development of the posts and continued to offer supervision and support as the posts became incorporated into the organisation. Just re-naming the posts would not have been enough or correct for the service or individual. Steering the process for occupational therapy has enabled a more successful integration of new ways of working and subsequent relationships.

Equally, the extended role most familiar to occupational therapists is that of care coordinator under the Care Programme Approach (CPA), which was introduced as the framework for the care of people with mental health needs in England (DH, 1990). Care coordination was designed to assess needs and provide relevant packages of care. It entailed a systematic assessment of individuals' health and social care needs, the appointment of an identified key worker, care plans, regular review and active involvement of service users in their care. Initially, the profession questioned whether the CPA coordinator role diluted the core skills of the profession or whether carrying out this role allowed occupational therapists credibility and standing within the multi-disciplinary team.

However, it is now common practice that occupational therapists carry out CPA coordinator roles and other generic functions, for example, on-call duties, work out of office hours and lead multi-disciplinary teams. As Ormston cited in Creek (2002, p. 176) notes occupational therapists adopt a number of roles generic to any mental health worker in a contemporary service context. In multi-disciplinary teams, they have to respond flexibly to a client-centred approach in which a number of generic skills are needed. Gaining clarity about the balancing of generic and specialist, core, acquired and required roles of occupational therapists is essential. Duncan (1999) argued that the quest for the uniqueness of occupational therapy can appear reminiscent of an adolescent identify crisis, and there is a danger that adopting a narrow construct of identity will lead to a prescriptive format and limited practice. He proposed the notion of shared skills and specialist skills as a way to conceptualise the profession's status.

Meeting the Challenge: A Strategy for the Allied Health Professions (DH, 2000b) set out how the role of allied health professions (AHP) could be developed in the future as a central element in delivering the NHS Plan. An important feature of this strategy was the creation of the post of consultant therapist whose core function would be expert clinical practice in addition to professional leadership, practice and service development; research and evaluation; and education and professional development. The focus of the consultant occupational therapist was about the delivery and practice of clinical care, tailored to local needs and based on local circumstances (COT, 2004). Craik and McKay (2003) welcomed the development of these posts and proposed that therapists would have to be proactive in their career plans to enable them to take the challenges offered by these posts. Targets for the number of posts to be established were issued but have not yet been fully achieved. However, some occupational therapy consultant posts have been developed and numbers have grown, if somewhat slowly.

In recent years, extended scope of practice and new ways of working have continued to challenge how and where occupational therapy is best placed. Currently, occupational therapists cannot prescribe, administer or supply medication, but it has been recommended that they be included in the Patient Group Directions. This would mean that, of the three methods of prescribing, occupational therapists could be potentially involved in-patient group direction (supply and administration) and supplementary prescribing (working with a doctor). Once again the College has provided briefing information on the scope of practice to date and is continually updating this as developments occur.

New ways of working

Linked to the new roles previously discussed are new ways of working. Government guidance once again highlights the need to review working activities and their intended outcome and to consider alternative methods of delivery such *New Ways of Working for Psychiatrists* (DH, 2005). It aimed to support and enable consultant psychiatrists to deliver effective and person-centred care concentrating on service users with the most complex needs enabling other members of the multi-disciplinary team to take on more responsibility. Therefore, new ways of working impact not only psychiatry but also nursing, psychology, social work and occupational therapy. Occupational therapists are now preparing their own document to reflect their specialist knowledge and skills in mental health for new or changing roles and responsibilities. This should not result in fundamentally changing what therapists do or the focus of intervention but should confirm occupational therapy as one of the five key professions in mental health.

Other influences

Occupational therapists are taking on more of an influencing role internally within organisations and externally in the current and wider mental health arena.

The College of Occupational Therapists has become more proactive in the area of policy development especially in mental health. Examples of this include the secondment of an occupational therapist to the Social Exclusion Unit, the development of the Mental Health Strategy (College of Occupational Therapists, 2006a) and the development of new ways of working guidance for occupational therapists.

Another significant national initiative that has influenced mental health policy and practice was the development of the National Institute for Clinical Excellence (NICE) for England and Wales in 1999. It is an independent organisation responsible for providing national guidance on promoting good health and preventing ill health. They produce three types of guidance: on public health, health technology and clinical practice. To date, completed clinical practice guidelines relating to mental health include those for anxiety, depression, depression in children and young people, eating disorders, obsessive compulsive disorders, post-traumatic stress disorder and schizophrenia.

Occupational therapists have contributed directly as representatives on the committees or as consultants developing the guidance. For example, occupational therapists working in eating disorders read the drafts and suggested amendments, largely centred on changing terminology, to reflect more of an occupational performance perspective. The College of Occupational Therapists also submitted evidence to the bipolar affective disorder guidelines relating to evidence of effective best practice. Individual occupational therapists have also commented on the consultations. Similarly, the College was also a registered stakeholder for the guidance developed on violence and aggression, emphasising the value of activity, time use and structuring and the use of therapeutic space.

Significantly, occupational therapists have played an influencing role in legislation; the revision of Mental Health Act (1983). Originally there was to be a new Mental Health Bill, but owing to robust opposition and lobbying from interested parties in the mental health field, the government decided to revise the existing act. Linked to this, are the proposed new roles of approved mental health practitioner (AMHP) and the clinical supervisor (likely to be called the responsible clinician).

Under the Mental Health Act (1983) compulsory detention of people with mental health problems requires a decision to be made by two medical officers and an approved social worker (ASW). In line with other efforts to modernise the workforce and a shortage of ASWs, it has been proposed to extend their role to other professions. It is unclear as to who will initially take up the role of an AMHP. Occupational therapists working in community mental health teams would most likely be considered for these roles along with their nursing colleagues.

Along with many colleagues who work in mental health, I believe that the inclusion of occupational therapists as professionals eligible to train as an AMHP will confer authority on their current clinical decisions to initiate a Mental Health Act assessment. Occupational therapists frequently initiate the process of assessment for detention, in their capacity as care coordinators, and in cases of team working such as assertive outreach, they are involved in the decision to embark on assessment and detention as an appropriate course of action. Occupational therapists have the requisite skills to take on this new role.

The second new role is that of the clinical supervisor or responsible clinician, which it is proposed will replace the responsible medical officer (RMO). Under the current legislation, the RMO is the position held by the consultant psychiatrist who is responsible for the detained patient. It is anticipated that the responsible clinician will be appointed in relation to the primary needs of the patient and will relate to the Mental Health Act amendment definition of treatment. This definition will ensure that care, facilitation and rehabilitation can be supervised by professionals other than medical personnel. In future, it will be considered good practice to have a responsible clinician of the most appropriate discipline to coordinate and hold responsibility of the patient's treatment package. This person could be an occupational therapist.

Not everyone in the profession agrees with the development of these new roles and new ways of working, criticising them as eroding professional skills and philosophies and the focus that occupational therapists bring to their work with service users. But the Mental Health Strategy (COT, 2006a) reinforces the need for therapists to remain current and be active in new ways of delivering services.

Conclusion

Current practice of occupational therapy in mental health is best summarised by the flavour presented in the College of Occupational Therapists Mental Health Strategy (2006). In essence, it suggests that occupational therapists will be the leaders in providing creative solutions for the activities and occupations in people's lives, thus playing a major role in the rehabilitation and recovery of individuals to lead the lives they choose to have for their well-being.

The future looks healthy and exciting presenting a great open door of opportunity for the profession. Occupational therapy is responding to new contexts but needs to be mindful of maintaining the values and ideals that underpin the profession whatever be the changing nature of mental health service provision. This needs to be done not only at national level but also by individual therapists, who need to engage with policy agenda and think through possible implications for their working practices. This means that therapists will have to actively consider new developments and contribute to the larger debate, overcoming their reliance on the profession to do this for them.

Equally important, therapists must not allow external policy alone to shape the future of the profession. Research and development within the profession, both in the UK and internationally, should also be fundamental to its future growth and direction.

In summary, the profession is

- involved in many of the government polices and initiatives both influencing the development of, and participating, in their implementation
- carrying out a wide variety of roles (both new and extended) in the mental health field in a variety of practice settings

- striving to keep occupation at the heart of practice
- working to be part of a flexible and adaptable workforce
- changing to meet changing demands and circumstances.

Questioning your practice

1. Where are occupational therapy skills best placed – practice or policy?
2. What are the key factors to think about in changing the occupational therapy workforce?
3. What key pieces of legislation have influenced your practice and why?

References

Allot P, Loganathan L, Fulford KWM (2002) Discovering Hope for Recovery from a British perspective: a review of a selection of Recovery Literature, implications for practice and systems change. International Innovations in Mental Health (special issue) *Canadian Journal of Community Mental Health, 21(2)*, 13–33.

College of Occupational Therapists (2003) *Briefing Paper: Mental Health Policy Implementation Guidelines, Support, Time and Recovery Workers.* London: College of Occupational Therapists.

College of Occupational Therapists (2004) *Briefing Paper: Consultant Occupational Therapists.* London: College of Occupational Therapists.

College of Occupational Therapists (2005) *Briefing Paper: Prescribing, Supply and Administration of Medicines and Occupational Therapists.* London: College of Occupational Therapists.

College of Occupational Therapists (2006a) *The Strategy for Occupational Therapy in Mental Health Services: Recovering Ordinary Lives.* London: College of Occupational Therapists.

College of Occupational Therapists (2006b) *Vocational Rehabilitation, Employment Opportunities and Condition Management: Draft Position Statement.* London: College of Occupational Therapists.

College of Occupational Therapists (2006c) *Extended Scope of Practice Briefing.* London: College of Occupational Therapists.

Craik C, Austin C, Chacksfield J, Richards G, Schell D (1998a) College of Occupational Therapists position paper on the way ahead for research, education and practice in mental health. *British Journal of Occupational Therapy, 61(9)*, 390–392.

Craik C, Chacksfield J, Richards G (1998b) A survey of occupational therapy practitioners in mental health. *British Journal of Occupational Therapy, 61(5)*, 227–233.

Craik C, McKay EA (2003) Consultant Therapists: recognising and developing expertise. *British Journal of Occupational Therapy, 66(8)*, 281–283.

Creek J (2002) *Occupational Therapy and Mental Health.* London: Churchill Livingstone.

Creek J (2003) *Occupational Therapy Defined as a Complex Intervention.* London: College of Occupational Therapists.

Department of Health (1990) *Caring for People, the CPA for People with a Mental Illness Referred to Specialist Mental Health Services.* Joint Health/Social Services Circular C(90)23/LASSL(90)11.

Department of Health (1999) *National Service Framework for Mental Health: Modern Standards and Service Models.* London: HMSO

Department of Health (2000a) *National Health Service Plan.* London: HMSO.

Department of Health (2000b) *Meeting the Challenge: A strategy for the Allied Health Professions*. London: HMSO.

Department of Health (2003a) *Mental Health Policy Implementation Guide: Support, Time and Recovery (STR) Worker*. London: HMSO.

Department of Health (2003b) *Fast Forwarding Primary Care Mental Health, Graduate Primary Care Mental Health Workers – Best Practice Guidance*. London: HMSO.

Department of Health (2004a) *The National Service Framework for Mental Health: Five Years On*. London: HMSO.

Department of Health (2004b) *Policy Implementation Guide. Community Development Workers for Black and Minority Ethnic Communities, Interim Guidance*. London: HMSO.

Department of Health (2005) *New Ways of Working for Psychiatrists: Enhancing Effective, Person Centred Services through New Ways of Working in Multidisciplinary Teams and Multi-Agency Contexts*. London: HMSO.

Department for Work and Pensions (2006) *A New Deal for Welfare: Empowering People to Work*. Command paper 6730.

Duncan E (1999) Occupational therapy in mental health: is it time to recognise that it has come of age? *British Journal of Occupational Therapy, 62(11)*, 521–522.

Great Britain: Parliament (1983) *Mental Health Act 1983*. London: HMSO.

Harries PA, Gilhooly K (2003) Generic and specialist occupational therapy casework in community mental health teams. *British Journal of Occupational Therapy, 66(3)*, 101–109.

Kings Fund (2006) *Grow Your Own: Creating the Conditions for Sustainable Workforce Development*. London: Kings Fund.

Mc Culloch A, Glover G, St John T (2003) The National Service Framework for Mental Health: past, present and future. *Mental Health Review, 8(4)*, 7–17.

Meeson B (1998a) Occupational therapy in community mental health, Part 1: intervention choice. *British Journal of Occupational Therapy, 61(1)*, 7–12.

Meeson B (1998b) Occupational therapy in community mental health, Part 2: factors influencing intervention choice. *British Journal of Occupational Therapy, 61(2)*, 57–62.

National Institute for Mental Health in England (2003) *Employment for People with Mental Health Problems*. London: Department of Health.

National Institute for Mental Health in England (2004a) *National Mental Health Workforce Strategy*. London: Department of Health.

National Institute for Mental Health in England (2004b) *The Ten Shared Essential Capabilities, A Framework for the Whole of the Mental Health Workforce*. London: Department of Health.

National Institute for Mental Health in England (2005) *Guiding statement on Recovery*. London: Department of Health.

National Social Inclusion Programme, National Institute for Mental Health in England (NIMHE), Care Services Improvement Partnership (CSIP)(2006). *Vocational Services for People with Severe Mental Health Problems: Commissioning Guidance*: London: Department of Health.

Office of the Deputy Prime Minister (2004) *Mental Health and Social Exclusion: Social Exclusion Unit Report*. London: HMSO.

Ormston C (1999) The National Service Framework for mental health: worth waiting for? *Occupational Therapy News, 7(12)*, 10–12.

Ormston C (2006) The underlying value base for occupational therapy practice – a constant in a changing environment. *Mental Health Occupational Therapy, 11(3)*, 102–103.

Rebeiro Gruhl KL (2005) Reflections on the recovery paradigm: should occupational therapists be interested? *Canadian Journal of Occupational Therapy, 72(2)*, 96–102.

Robdale N (2004) Vocational Rehabilitation: the enable, employment and retention scheme, a new approach. *British Journal of Occupational Therapy, 67(10)*, 457–460.

Sainsbury Centre for Mental Health (1997) *Pulling Together: The Future Roles and Training Needs for Mental Health Staff*. London: Sainsbury Centre for Mental Health.

Sainsbury Centre for Mental Health (2003) *A Mental Health Workforce for the Future*. London: Sainsbury Centre for Mental Health.

Sainsbury Centre for Mental Health (2005) *Defining a Good Mental Health Service – A Discussion Paper*. London: Sainsbury Centre for Mental Health.

3 Cultural sensitivity in context

Kee Hean Lim

Personal narrative

Ah Seng was a frequent visitor around our neighbourhood, and he would often be found asking for money or small jobs to do in return for some financial reward. I was 6 years old when I became aware of his visits, and I was intrigued by who he was and where he came from. I discovered that my father knew him. This took place in a housing estate of British colonial homes in Singapore in the 1970s. My father was the chief pharmacist at the psychiatric institution in Singapore, Woodbridge Hospital, near where we lived. Ah Seng was a patient in a long-term rehabilitation ward; as he was not considered to be a risk to others, he enjoyed the freedom to roam the surrounding area.

This triggered my interest in him and the other patients, and led me during my school holidays to spend time with my father at the hospital. The seeds were sown of my journey into mental health and my subsequent career as an occupational therapist. I recalled observing the industrial therapy, social and creative groups that the patients engaged in. I noticed that they demonstrated a real sense of industry in these activities, appearing to derive satisfaction from their involvement. I did not realise then that it was occupational therapy.

My journey began in 1989 at the London School of Occupational Therapy (now Brunel University) in the UK. I vividly remember my first weeks in the UK, where I was struck by the distinct socio-cultural differences and perspectives. Certain patterns of behaviour that in Singapore would be frowned upon were esteemed in this new environment. Questioning individuals in authority, such as lecturers, and articulating ideas instead of speaking only when you were spoken to were both new and unsettling. These differences highlighted the importance of appreciating the complexity of how individuals are shaped by their socio-cultural context and lived experience (Lim & Iwama, 2006).

My first occupational therapy post in 1992 was in a secure psychiatric unit in a large London mental hospital. This experience was daunting and intriguing. The clients were unwell and were detained as there was a high risk of violence. However, the containing nature of the ward and the skills and qualities of some staff appeared to minimise incidents and created a therapeutic milieu in this potentially hostile environment. What was notable was the disproportionate number of black young men on the ward – a phenomenon replicated throughout the hospital.

Cultural sensitivity, in this context, is my passion and research interest. This includes culturally sensitive practice, socio-cultural construction of occupational therapy and occupation, social inclusion and recovery of mental health service users and the Kawa 'River' Model.

Introduction

This chapter will clarify the key terms used and explore the evolving socio-cultural contexts. This will be followed by views of cross-cultural mental health and will conclude by exploring culturally sensitive practice and professional and personal imperatives. Although focused primarily on the UK, the issues raised and strategies suggested in addressing cultural sensitivity are relevant internationally.

Clarification of key terms

There is confusion around the concepts of culture, minority ethnic groups, cultural sensitivity and competency as these terms are defined and understood in a variety of ways (Dillard et al., 1992; Fitzgerald et al., 1997; Awaad, 2003). The terms client and service user will be used interchangeably.

Culture

Wells and Black (2000, p. 279) defined culture 'as a set of values, beliefs, traditions, norms, artefacts and customs that is shared by a group or society'. Whilst Hasselkus (2002, p. 42) stated that culture consists of 'patterns of values, beliefs, symbols, perceptions and learnt behaviours shared by members of a group and passed on from one generation to another'. What is significant and valuable to a particular cultural group may not be shared by the majority population or wider society (Lim, 2006a). Culture is evolving and dynamic, and therefore assumptions made about any cultural group, and their responses, may alter with time (Awaad, 2003; Chaing & Carlson, 2003).

Lim and Iwama (2006) proposed that a selection of ethnically diverse individuals who are socialised within a common community may subscribe to an agreed set of values and principles despite their racial differences. They warned of the dangers of racial assumptions and stereotypes that influence and bias interpretations. They suggested that information gained before interviewing and assessing clients, although valuable, must be verified and supplemented by the clients, as they provide the best reference point for their cultural beliefs, needs and preferences (Lim, 2001; Tribe, 2002). The provision of culturally sensitive care involves an appreciation of the socio-cultural context and cultural influences that shape individuals' identity, perspective and lived experience (Keating, 2006). Acknowledging, affirming and valuing clients' perspectives are important in validating their personal experiences (Hocking & Whiteford, 1995; Howarth & Jones, 1999; McGruder, 2003).

Minority ethnic communities

Wells and Black (2000, p. 282) define minority ethnic communities as 'a group of persons who, because of their physical or cultural characteristics, are singled out from others in the society in which they live, for differential and unequal treatment and who regard themselves as objects of collective discrimination'. Bhugra and Bahl (1999) exclude national minorities such as the Scottish, Northern Irish and Welsh, who, despite their equal rights, have distinct cultural traditions and values, and argue that the current provision of services for them takes into account their specific needs. However, this view may not be shared by these respective communities who may feel that their cultural traditions and values are not sufficiently acknowledged (Leavey, 1999).

A study of occupational therapy students at Brunel University explored issues of ethnicity, race, culture, health and well-being. The majority of white (English) students felt uncomfortable and struggled to identify their own ethnicity: they had never thought about themselves in these terms and found the task difficult. In contrast, students from minority ethnic groups had no such difficulties – identifying issues relating to their ethnicity, race and being different were frequently reinforced within their daily lives, through experiences of discrimination and prejudice (Reynolds & Lim, 2005).

Cultural sensitivity and competence

The key to cultural sensitivity and competence involves the willingness of practitioners to explore the meaning of culture and to acquire knowledge about cultural issues, including their personal bias (Dillard *et al.*, 1992; Wells & Black, 2000; Reynolds & Lim, 2005). Cultural competence cannot be achieved by completing a course of study. Wells and Black (2000) suggest that it requires self-awareness, a cultural knowledge base, an ability to access relevant information, learning to interact with others with sensitivity and respect, developing appropriate practice and an ability to evaluate personal performance and outcomes.

The evolving socio-cultural context

Increased globalisation has fostered the freedom to travel, work and live abroad and has promoted the consequential cross-cultural exchange of narratives, knowledge and experiences. The Office for National Statistics (2001) indicated that 5.29 million people, representing 8.9 % of the UK population, are from minority ethnic groups. The increased diversity is found throughout the country, although minority ethnic groups make up a significant proportion of populations in Leicester, Manchester, Glasgow and Bradford (Office for National Statistics, 2001). In London, 29% of the population is from minority ethnic groups, and in some communities, this figure rises to over 50% (King's Fund, 2003).

The recent expansion of the EU has also increased the population diversity within the UK. A view that the UK is overpopulated and overwhelmed by immigrants is perpetuated by inaccurate and provocative reports in the media (Trivedi, 2002). These negative views extend to refugees and people seeking asylum and have the potential to prejudice perceptions of both these groups, with some believing that those seeking refuge in the UK are economic migrants rather than genuine refugees. This has an adverse effect on refugees trying to settle and integrate into the UK. However, such myths are discredited when the Office for National Statistics (2005) indicates that over a thousand British citizens are migrating from the UK daily.

Assimilation and integration into mainstream society requires that migrants and refugees go beyond existing; they must be able to live, work and contribute and have the freedom to be, belong and become without fear, exclusion or discrimination (Reynolds & Lim, 2005). This is impossible when migrants and refugees are segregated in deprived areas with other social excluded members of society (Lim, 2005; Smith, 2005). Conflict and jealousy arise when the majority population perceive that their already limited resources are being siphoned away by migrant groups. Issues of social and occupational injustice, loss of opportunity, intolerance and prejudice can lead to further discrimination and even greater social exclusion (Whiteford, 2000; Wilcock, 2006).

With prejudice and injustice, social inclusion and integration are unlikely to occur. This situation can be compounded by mental illness. The Social Exclusion Unit (Office of the Deputy Prime Minister, 2004) indicates that refugees and minority ethnic groups with a mental illness are the most excluded people in the UK. Thus, the promotion of social inclusion in enabling individuals to participate fully in society, enjoying the same opportunities and engaging in daily activities of their choice, becomes an impossible dream. This is reinforced by Smith (2005), who highlights the shortage of social capital, opportunities and resources required to support the educational, health and social needs of these groups.

National recognition of discrimination, racism, inequality and lack of cultural safety led to policies and standards to address these issues within health and social care (DH, 1999; DH, 2000; Office of the Deputy Prime Minister, 2004) and particularly in Delivering Race Equality in Mental Health Consultation Document (DH, 2003), which all reflect the importance of eliminating the problems of cultural insensitivity and promoting access, choice, opportunity and equality.

High-profile inquiries conducted by, MacPherson (1999) and Blofeld (2003) highlighted the poor levels of care and discriminatory treatment received by black and minority ethnic (BME) service users, and led to the Delivering Race Equality in Mental Health (DRE) Action Plan (DH, 2005a). This 5-year plan aims to achieve equality and to tackle discrimination in mental health services by outlining objectives, initiatives and targets for mental health services. To support the plan, a national steering group has been commissioned to ensure that current and future mental health practitioners are equipped with relevant cultural knowledge and skills to work competently with a diverse range of clients in equitable and culturally sensitive ways.

UK mental health ethnicity statistics

Wilson and Francis (1997) noted that African, African-Caribbean and Irish people were over-represented in psychiatric hospitals and Irish people were over-represented in alcohol services in the UK. Browne (1997) further found that African and African-Caribbean people were more likely to be detained under the Mental Health Act. The Sainsbury Centre for Mental Health (SCMH) (2000) and a systematic review by Bhui *et al.* (2003) noted that the lack of cultural sensitivity and appropriateness of existing assessments may contribute to misdiagnosis and disparities in treatment options available to BME service users. More recently, the Healthcare Commission Census (DH, 2005b) reported that BME service users encountered greater involvement of the police in their referrals and higher rates of physical restraint than other patient groups. Central to these inequalities was the failure of staff to appreciate the individuals' lived experience (Lim, 2001; Trivedi, 2002). Mind (2002) reported that, although black men represent 1% of the UK population, they are ten times more likely to be diagnosed with a mental health problem. They are more likely to receive physical treatments, be given atypical medication and are less likely to be referred for talking therapies; additionally they make up 16% of those detained in one high-security hospital.

In contrast, such groups as Chinese and South Asians (including Sikhs) are under-represented in mental health services (Bhui *et al.*, 2003). This may be due to genetics or increased resilience to mental health problems or, conversely, that they experience greater difficulty in accessing help or avoid mental health services (Lim, 2001). Additional efforts must be made to understand this phenomenon to ensure that people from these groups are not disadvantaged

Providing culturally appropriate food, having information in different languages and interpretation services are a start, but are not enough to address intolerance of religious beliefs and customs, discrimination and inflexibility in making adjustments to respect the values and needs of individuals (Lim, 2001).

The death of Stephen Lawrence, a black teenager in East London in 1993, led to a public inquiry that concluded that institutional racism, defined as 'a collective failure of an organisation to provide an appropriate and professional service to people because of their colour, culture or ethnic origins', existed within public services in UK society (MacPherson, 1999, p. 4262-i). Such discrimination can be overt or covert and is detected within the attitudes, behaviours and processes of an organisation. Although unintentional, it may be demonstrated through unwitting prejudice, thoughtlessness and racist stereotyping, which disadvantages minority ethnic people. Reflecting these findings, Greenwood *et al.* (2000) and Secker and Harding (2002) explored the in-patient experiences of service users from Asian, African and African-Caribbean backgrounds who reported a loss of control, experience of overt and implicit racism, unhelpful relationships with some staff and a lack of therapeutic groups and activities during their admission.

The independent inquiry into the death of David Bennett (Blofeld, 2003) stressed the failure of the National Health Service (NHS) to tackle institutional racism and the excessive use of physical restraints and recommended that all staff receive cultural awareness and sensitivity training. As it is difficult to separate the attitudes and practices of employees from their organisation that influences their actions (SCMH, 2002), occupational therapists need to examine the professional philosophies and principles within their practice (Lim, 2005) to ensure inclusive, cultural by sensitive and non-discriminatory services to clients.

Inequalities in power

Central to the process of involvement is the power to influence decisions affecting one's treatment, health and social requirements. However, despite national initiatives to promote greater service user involvement, collaboration is often superficial (Trivedi, 1999; Keating, 2006). Trivedi (2002) proposed that staff are vested with more power than clients and this inequality is more than even the most confident, skilled and empowered client could overcome. To lessen this inequality, staff need to ensure that clients are enabled to influence their own goals and treatment (Hinkin & Schresheim, 1994; Lim, 2005).

At a societal level, the negative impact of mental health services, as experienced by certain communities, perpetuates the belief that these services are part of a larger system that subjugates and restricts freedom of choice and lifestyle (Mintzberg, 1983; Trivedi, 2002). These minority ethnic groups may perceive that the mental health system fulfils a more sinister role of social control, enforcement and exclusion (Keating, 2006). The following example captures this view.

Cross-cultural mental health perspectives

The cross-cultural interpretation of mental illness may be different from Western conceptualisation that frames individual's experience into categories of ill health. Diagnosis is important, as treatment is centred on identifying and counteracting the problem (Masi, 1992; Lim, 2001). This contrasts with the non-Western perspective, where mental ill health may be attributed to a failure to maintain life balance or a consequence of witchcraft or incurring a curse (Helman, 2000). This view negates the importance of adhering to a medication regime, and a visit to a healer or maintaining a balance through traditional remedies may be reasoned to be more effective.

Non-Western perspectives of health and well-being

Effective practice in a multi-cultural context requires an appreciation of how individuals understand their world, their philosophy and what they perceive as meaningful. In the UK, Western perspectives and priorities are dominant. Although cultural and philosophical differences may not be an issue when working with individuals from a similar background, they may be potential hurdles when working cross-culturally. Diverse individuals and communities require occupational therapists to examine alternative views and experiences (Iwama, 2003; Lim, 2004a). Although these perspectives are not totally exclusive to each group or shared by all its members, they are generally shared by individuals within Western and non-Western societies. These differences are identified in Table 3.1.

The Western perspective of health and well-being purports a reductionist and scientific view; in contrast, the non-Western, holistic perspective focuses on inter-related factors contributing to the difficulties experienced. Health and well-being are not the absence of illness, but equilibrium is achieved through all aspects of the individual's life (Lim & Iwama, 2006). It is a cyclical process with inter-related components connected to a larger whole. Acceptance and contemplation are natural and necessary for recovery and the maintenance of health is dependent on balance and harmony between the inter-related components (Henley & Schott, 1999; Servan-Schreiber, 2004). So, health and well-being are not achieved through discovering and eradicating a single identifiable problem but through the individual's ability to be in rhythm with societal and natural forces and maintaining a body, mind, soul and spiritual cohesion (Iwama, 2003).

In Western societies, where personal autonomy and independence are highly esteemed, the individual is important. The non-Western view is on collective interest and agreement, visualising the self as a component of a larger collective whole (Henley & Schott, 1999; Lim & Iwama, 2006). Maintaining harmony and unity are priorities in cultures where personal autonomy, independence and choice are not accorded the same status (Helman, 2000). The minority ethnic client, perceived as unassertive or indecisive, may be delaying a decision until family or community can be consulted (Lim, 2001). The Western world is characterised by pressures that require people to be doing, whereas the Eastern view expounds the virtues of

Table 3.1 Western and non-Western perspectives of health and well-being.

Western perspectives	Non-Western perspectives
Reductionist	Holist
Individualism and personal autonomy	Collectivism and harmony
Scientific analysis and problem solving	Awareness and contemplation
Control and doing	Acceptance and being
Domination	Balance

Source: From Lim and Iwama (2006). With permission.

contemplation, stillness and being, which are more important than doing; achievement is attained through contemplation rather than engagement (Lim & Iwama, 2006). The client who perceives illness as a consequence of an imbalance may seek alternative solutions beyond the medical model. As the UK and other Western countries have become multi-cultural societies, occupational therapists must be sensitive to the cultural interpretations of health and illness and consider their clients on many levels (Lim, 2001; Lim & Iwama, 2006).

Culturally sensitive practice: professional imperatives and personal strategies

Communication is the first step in the interaction between client and therapist, but this can be difficult if people do not speak the same language. Interpreters must speak the correct dialect as not all individuals from a particular ethnic background, cultural group or country use the same one. Not all health terms can be translated into the client's language, and phrasing questions accurately to elicit information can be problematic. If the word stress does not have a clear translation, it may be easier to ask about the symptoms of stress. Within some cultures, somatic symptoms may be a more culturally acceptable way of communicating psychological distress (Lim, 2001).

Central to occupational therapy is client-centred practice (COT, 2005). This requires the ability to examine personal, cultural and ethnic influences and their impact on values, beliefs and prejudices towards those encountered in practice (Wells & Black, 2000; McGruder, 2003; Lim, 2004a; Reynolds & Lim, 2005). Levy *et al.* (1998) warned against stereotyping, where one piece of information about an individual such as age, gender or race may generate inferences about all other aspects of that person. Gross (2001) states that personal/social values influence relationships but should not be imposed on clients and their carers. The consequence of presuming that occupational therapists know what is most beneficial for clients becomes apparent when they are labelled non-compliant, demotivated, disgruntled or simply absent from treatment (Wetherell, 1996; Lim, 2001). There may be different reasons for their behaviour. A lack of skill or awareness on the part of the professional, in imposing inappropriate or culturally insensitive practices, may elicit the undesired response. Sensitivity to the cultural dimensions of each client is needed to form a therapeutic partnership (McGruder, 2003).

The World Federation of Occupational Therapists' Position Statement on Human Rights (2006, p. 1) states that 'people have the right to participate in a range of occupations that enable them to flourish, fulfil their potential and experience satisfaction in a way consistent with their culture and beliefs'.

The challenge for occupational therapists is to cross the cultural divide, establish contact and partnerships with individuals and communities that are marginalised, socially excluded or occupationally deprived, to enable opportunities for equal participation (Lim, 2005). Christie (2003) identified strategies to support culturally and socially inclusive service delivery. These include equipping clients through skills development and working with them to ensure their involvement and influence in all aspects of service delivery.

Whiteford (2000) proposed that occupational therapists should become agents of change, in adopting an occupational perspective that considers the occupational needs of individuals within society. Townsend (1999) and Wilcock (2006) challenge occupational therapists to invest time and energy in influencing social and institutional structures to review their policies and standards to support the specific needs of those who are deprived, excluded or discriminated against, and to confront negative attitudes and to promote social inclusion. Kronenberg *et al.* (2005) emphasised the importance of occupational therapists being engaged in political activities of daily living in supporting and influencing political, economic, environmental, social, cultural and systemic change. They acknowledged the power of professionals to advocate on behalf of clients and communities that are marginalised. Change begins with vision and passion to see minority ethnic clients and communities experiencing improvement in their treatment by health and social care services. There must be a collective effort and commitment to make a difference for all groups within society (Reynolds &Lim, 2005).

Ensuring cultural sensitivity, competence and equality in practice is enshrined in the profession's code of ethics (COT, 2005; WFOT, 2006). It requires occupational therapists to account for the diverse needs, values and perspectives of clients, but this intent must be implemented and evaluated to move from rhetoric to action. Most frameworks and models of occupational therapy, which reflect a Western stance, influence this commitment. Although they facilitate understanding and work with individuals, their value is limited cross-culturally (Lim, 2004a). Competing worldviews challenge the adequacy of existing models and frameworks to explain occupational phenomena for all (Iwama, 2003; Chaing & Clarson, 2003).

The Kawa 'River' Model is the first occupational therapy model developed from the East and it provides a radical perspective of how occupation and individual self is conceptualised (see Table 3.2). It arose as a consequence of Japanese occupational therapists' frustration with the utility of Western models and concepts that were not resonant with their personal or client's socio-cultural experiences (Iwama, 2006). Importantly, the Kawa Model indicates a major change from Western concepts and ideas, promoting the importance of discourse and validation of alternative perspectives (Lim & Iwama, 2006). Distinctively, it is devoid of linear structures, line, boxes and technical jargon. It is infused with a naturalistic and holistic perspective of life, health and well-being, and adopts the metaphor of a river – Kawa means river in Japanese. Each individual is perceived as having a unique personal river, which symbolises his or her life journey – the upstream of the river represents the past and the downstream represents the future. Personal health and well-being is expressed by the free and unrestricted flow of the river, whilst life difficulties, problems, barriers, environmental, financial and social constraints are symbolised by rocks and the restrictive river bank (Lim & Iwama, 2006).

Table 3.2 Five key components of the Kawa 'River' Model.

Water

Water represents the client's life energy and health

Water is flexible and is shaped by its container (experience, circumstances)

The river can flow fully, dry up and change directions

Water can be clear or be in a muddy state

Riversides and bottom

Represent the client's physical and social environment and human resources

Family, healthcare professionals, school, workplace, culture and society can shape one's
environment

Rocks

Represent the client's life difficulties

They block and slow down the water flow

Disease, symptoms and daily life challenges are represented as rocks

Driftwood

Represents the client's attributes, values, character and experiences that can work
positively or negatively (assets and liabilities)

Driftwood can either further block the water flow or bump the rocks away enhancing the flow

Spaces

Represent the client's natural healing power, potential and include abilities and positive
points

Enhancing the client's inner ability and maximising opportunities is one of the major
aspects of occupational therapy

Case Study 3.1   Application of the Kawa Model

Krishna is 34 years old and unmarried. He lives with his supportive family, who can be overcon-
cerned at times. Krishna has been diagnosed with schizophrenia and has a 15-year history of
mental illness and relapse. He has an intermittent work history but enjoys using computers and
is currently keen to do some voluntary work. He is sociable with a strong and supportive network of friends and family. However, he has poor concentration and self-care skills. He receives
long-term sickness benefit. He is currently compliant with his medication and regularly attends
his appointments with his occupational therapists and community psychiatric nurse.

To illustrate the Kawa Model, Krishna's mental health difficulties are presented
as pictorial representations of his river at a point in time (Figure 3.1) and how
occupational therapy may be used to help him overcome his difficulties (Box 3.1).

The author's experience of utilising the Kawa Model has reinforced the opinion
that the concept of a river, representing a life journey, is simple and understood by

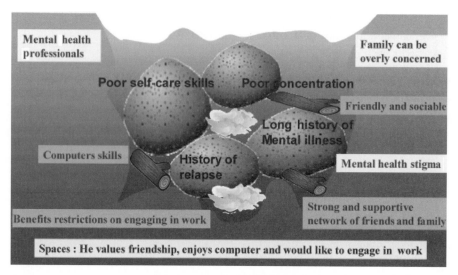

Figure 3.1 Krishna's Kawa River.

Box 3.1   Krishna's occupational therapy intervention.

Water

■ The aim of occupational therapy is to maximise Krishna's life-flow. This will involve reducing and removing elements that presently impede his river's flow and maximising existing channels or spaces where his water currently flows.

Rocks

■ Identify the rocks, their relative size and location. Determine with Krishna and his family which obstacles are most troublesome to him.
■ Krishna and his family report that he is not able to look after his self-care.

Manipulate the rocks

■ Reduce the obstacles by providing help with self-care skills including personal grooming, laundry and meal preparation. Monitor his mental health status. Work on increasing his concentration skills through participation in relevant/meaningful activities, such as computer skills training.

Spaces/channels

■ Identify current and potential spaces, and their location, paying attention to the context surrounding the flow.
■ Determine which spaces are most important and meaningful to Krishna.

Box 3.1 *Continued*

Maximising the spaces

■ Promote his inner strength, interest, abilities and skills. These may include: work preparation training, exploring voluntary work, attending the local sports centre to meet new friends and build stamina, and working on personal CV.

River bed and sides

Widen the riversides and deepen the river bottom

■ Consult with benefits advisor to assess Krishna's benefit status in relation to paid voluntary work.
■ Provide support for Krishna and his family in terms of regular family meetings to help the family understand Krishna's condition and his desire to engage in voluntary work, and to do more for himself.
■ Facilitate a process to involve his whole professional team and family in supporting his engagement in voluntary work, his social interests and computer skills training.

Driftwood

■ Identify aspects of character and attributes, and materials that may act as assets or liabilities in the Krishna's life-flow. Determine Krishna's cultural and social context, toward an understanding of factors that will help or hinder his occupational well-being.

Utilise the driftwood

■ Enhance the positive aspects of his character and attributes: friendliness, desire for voluntary work, build on his computer skills, getting his family to support his desire to get fit, socialise and engage in work, etc.

clients (Lim, 2006b). In this example, Krishna was immediately able to comprehend it. He gained understanding of how his personal river reflected his life journey and how the rocks in his river were representations of his difficulties. He was able to focus on his assets and strengths (driftwood and spaces) in terms of his friendly and sociable disposition, his previous computer skills and his desire to engage in work and examine how these positive aspects could be harnessed in overcoming his difficulties. During the process, Krishna identified the rocks within his river as representing his poor concentration, his history of mental illness and periods of relapse.

The initial depiction of his river allowed discussion around his views of his difficulties and what his family identified as an additional rock, his self-care needs, which he had not perceived to be a concern (Lim, 2006b). The pictorial representation of Krishna's river facilitated examination of how his priorities and concerns were different from those of his family. Within the family sessions, Krishna's parents were able to appreciate the issues that Krishna perceived as barriers restricting his recovery and to understand how they might assist him in achieving his future goals.

The Kawa Model visualises the individual in the wider context and examines how the familial, social, environmental, professional, political and economic contextual influences may support or limit the journey to health and recovery. It also provides a framework for the occupational therapist and client to focus on the holistic interplay of strengths, difficulties, assets, circumstances and pressures that may impact on the individual (Lim & Iwama, 2006). The pictorial image that includes the needs as well as the strengths, assets and innate potential of the individual client to recover is unique to the Kawa Model. This visual quality promotes greater understanding and clarity for clients especially those with learning difficulties, children and those with limited literacy who might otherwise struggle to understand occupational therapy concepts. Thus, they can be more active in determining their own intervention (Lim, 2006b).

The Kawa Model does not possess a range of standardised measurements, but abides by the principle that the most culturally appropriate and sensitive assessments and interventions must be selected in all clinical situations (Iwama, 2005a; Lim & Iwama, 2006).

Research and use of the Kawa Model is limited at present in the UK and Europe but is gaining momentum. In Japan, where it first evolved, it has been used more extensively and there are over 800 case studies across the diverse spectrum of occupational therapy (Iwama, 2006). Current research is focused on examining the utility and development of the Kawa Model in the wider international and transcultural context. It is currently included within several occupational therapy educational curricula including the European occupational therapy master's programme and continues to generate discourse and global interest (Iwama, 2006).

Within the UK, occupational therapists working with older people, those with multiple sclerosis, mental health and cardiac care have began to utilise the Kawa Model (Iwama, 2006). An English language Web site and discussion forum has recently been established (www.kawamodel.com) to promote discourse around the relevance and appropriateness of the Kawa Model transculturally.

Outcome measurement and evidence-based practice

Outcome measurement and evidence-based practice are important in establishing the effectiveness of occupational therapy; however, therapists should not lose sight of whose outcomes they are measuring and whose health they are trying to promote (Lim, 2004a). The use of standardised assessments to assess clients and evaluate intervention raises several questions for those providing culturally sensitive care. The selection and use of outcome measures are guided by professional opinion and may represent the dominant discourse of the therapist or service, reflecting their outlook of health and well-being rather than that of the client (Iwama, 2005b; WFOT, 2006). Frequently, evidence is limited to easily measured end-points and compared against universal standards and may not actually reflect the perception of the client.

The majority of occupational therapy standardised measures have been derived from models of practice, and they may not apply to people of cultures different from the context in which they were developed. The appropriateness, utility and validity of these measures, beyond their original socio-cultural contexts, are limited (Lim & Iwama, 2006). The emphasis on standardised measures may conflict with the commitment to listen to the individuals' narrative, acknowledge their experience and understand their concerns. This appreciation of the client is essential in the delivery of culturally sensitive care and in enabling engagement in meaningful occupation. (Lim, 2004b; WFOT, 2006).

Ultimately, standardised assessments and outcome measures must be validated and verified for cultural safety, sensitivity and appropriateness for use with minority ethnic clients. In the meantime, to counteract the inherent bias, measures may be adapted appropriately or supplemented with additional narratives from the client.

Promoting mental health

Moving beyond intervention, Wilcock (2006) suggested that occupational therapists have a significant role in promoting health and well-being through engagement in meaningful occupation. However, this can only occur if the barriers that exclude service users from engaging and participating in their local communities are challenged and removed (Whiteford, 2000). Partnership working with minority ethnic communities aimed at reducing stigma and discrimination may assist the promotion of positive and inclusive mental health. Although this was recognised in the UK (DH, 1999), Sortland (2006) in a review of health and social care policies on promoting mental health indicated few specific standards aimed at addressing the needs of minority ethnic communities.

Education and training

Having occupational therapists that are culturally competent requires education and training. Lim's (2004b) study of 15 newly qualified occupational therapists from eight UK Universities indicated disparities in the amount and quality of culture awareness in the curriculum. Therefore, cultural competence must be as integral to the pre-registration education curriculum as other key occupational therapy concepts (WFOT. 2006, p. 2).

Delivering Race and Equality in Mental Health Programmes (2005) should promote cultural sensitivity and competence. Students and practitioners from all professions will have access to consistent education to assist them in the three stage process of undertaking personal examination and reflection, knowledge acquisition and skills training to become fully equipped to practise competently with a diverse spectrum of clients. This is especially important for therapists moving to a new geographical location where they may encounter people from different backgrounds. They should be proactive in seeking to understand these communities.

Summary

Promoting cultural sensitivity in practice begins with an acceptance that the client's interests and needs are of paramount importance. The appreciation of the client's unique socio-cultural context and lived experience enhances client-centred and culturally appropriate care. Clear communication, non-judgemental attitude and respect for the cultural and ethnic beliefs of clients are all important. The assessments, models and interventions used should be verified for diverse range of clients encountered in practice.

The influence of professional culture and the personal values of the therapist must be continually revisited and examined. Forging partnerships and collaboration is essential to enhancing client, carer and community involvement. Ultimately, the enhancement of cultural sensitivity demands listening, acknowledging, respecting and working with clients as equal partners in moving towards the improvement of their mental health.

Epilogue

Later, having practised as an occupational therapist in the UK, I returned to Singapore and visited the occupational therapy department at Woodbridge Hospital. Despite a gap of 25 years since our first encounter, I noticed a familiar individual working within the hospital dispensary. Here was a much older Ah Seng living in a supported home in the community and now engaged in supported employment as a part-time dispensary assistant in the hospital.

Questioning your Practice

1. How does my current practice reflect and fulfil the cultural needs and requirements of the clients with whom I work?
2. How does my practice translate cross-culturally?
3. In what ways is my practice influenced by organisational and professional philosophy, culture, priorities and structures?

References

Awaad T (2003) Culture, cultural competency and occupational therapy: A review of the literature. *British Journal of Occupational Therapy, 66(8)*, 356–362.

Bhugra D, Bahl V (1999) *Ethnicity: An Agenda for Mental Health.* London: Royal College of Psychiatrists.

Bhui K, Stansfeld S, Hull S (2003) Ethnic variations in pathways to and use of specialist mental health services in the UK: Sytematic review. *British Journal of Psychiatry, 182(2)*, 105–116.

Blofeld J (2003) *Independent Inquiry into the Death of David Bennett*. Norwich: Norfolk, Suffolk & Cambridgeshire Strategic Health Authority.

Browne D (1997) *Black People and Sectioning*. London: Little Rock Publishing.

Chaing M, Carlson G (2003) Occupational therapy in multicultural contexts: issues and strategies. *British Journal of Occupational Therapy*, 66(12), 559–566.

Christie Y (2003) *Black Spaces Project: A Report of Seven Black Voluntary Sector Projects*. London: Mental Health Foundation.

College of Occupational Therapists (2005) *Code of Ethics and Professional Conduct*. London: COT.

Department of Health (1999) *National Service Frameworks for Mental Health*. London: HMSO.

Department of Health (2000) *National Health Service Plan*. London: HMSO.

Department of Health (2003) *Delivering Race Equality in Mental Health: Consultation document*. London: HMSO.

Department of Health (2005a) *Delivering Race Equality in Mental Health Care: An Action Plan for Reform Inside and Outside Services and the Government's Response to the Independent Inquiry into the Death of David Bennett*. London: DH HMSO.

Department of Health (2005b) *The Healthcare Commission Census*. London: HMSO.

Dillard PA, Andonian L, Flores O, Lai L, MacRae A, Shakir M (1992) Culturally competent occupational therapy in a diversely populated mental health setting. *American Journal of Occupational Therapy, 46(8)*, 721–726.

Fitzgerald MH, Mullavey-O'Byrne C, Clemson L (1997) Cultural issues from practice. *Australian Occupational Therapy Journal, (44)*, 1–21.

Greenwood N, Hussain F, Burns T, Raphael F (2000) Asian inpatient and carer views of mental health care. *Journal of Mental Health, 9(4)*, 397–408.

Gross R (2001) Psychology: *The Science of Mind and Behaviour* (4th edn). London: Hodder & Stoughton.

Hasselkus BR (2002) *The Meaning of Everyday Occupation*. Thorofare NJ: Slack.

Helman CG (2000) *Culture, Difference and Healthcare*. Oxford: Butterworth Scientific.

Henley A, Schott J (1999) *Culture, Religion and Patient Care in a Multi-ethnic Society*. London: Age Concern Books.

Hinkin TR, Schriesheim CA (1994) An examination of subordinate-perceived relationships between leader reward and punishment behaviour and leader bases of power. *Human Relations, 47(7)*, 779–795.

Hocking C, Whiteford G (1995) Multiculturalism in occupational therapy: a time of reflection on core values. *Australian Occupational Therapy Journal, 42(4)*, 172–175.

Howarth A, Jones D (1999) Transcultural occupational therapy in the UK. *British Journal of Occupational Therapy, 62(10)*, 451–458.

Iwama M (2003) Towards culturally relevant epistemology in occupational therapy. *American Journal of Occupational Therapy, 57(5)*, 582–588.

Iwama M (2005a) The Kawa (river) Model; Nature, life flow & the power of culturally relevant occupational therapy. In: F Kronenberg, SA Algado, N Pollard (eds) *Occupational Therapy Without Borders – Learning from the Spirit of Survivors*. Edinburgh: Elsevier Churchill Livingstone, 213–227.

Iwama M (2005b) Situated meaning: An issue of culture, inclusion and occupational therapy. In: F Kronenberg, SA Algado, N Pollard (eds) *Occupational Therapy Without Borders – Learning from the Spirit of Survivors*. Edinburgh: Elsevier Churchill Livingstone, 127–139.

Iwama M (2006) *The Kawa River Model: Culturally Relevant Occupational Therapy*. Edinburgh: Elsevier Churchill Livingstone.

Keating F (2006) Breaking the spiral of oppression: racism and race equality in the mental health system. In: C Jackson, K Hill (eds). *Mental Health Today: A Handbook*. London: Pavilion.

King's Fund (2003) *London's Mental Health*. London: King's Fund.

Kronenberg F, Algado SA, Pollard N (2005) *Occupational Therapy Without Borders – Learning from the Spirit of Survivors*. Edinburgh: Churchill Livingstone.

Leavey G (1999) Suicide and Irish migrants in Britain: Identity and integration. *International Review of Psychiatry, 11(2–3)*, 168–172.

Levy S, Stroessner S, Dweck C (1998) Stereotype formation and endorsement: the role of implicit theories. *Journal of Personality & Social Psychology, 74(6)*, 1421–1436.

Lim KH (2001) A guide to providing culturally sensitive and appropriate occupational therapy assessments and interventions. *Mental Health Occupational Therapy Magazine, 6(2)*, 26–29.

Lim KH (2004a) Occupational therapy in multicultural contexts. *British Journal of Occupational Therapy, 67(1)*, 49–50.

Lim KH (2004b) Building a future together: Enabling and equipping occupational therapists to be culturally competent. Poster presented at the 24th September 2004 European Occupational Therapy Congress, Athens, Greece.

Lim KH (2005) Partnership, involvement and inclusion. *Mental Health Occupational Therapy, 10(1)*, 22–24.

Lim KH (2006a) The Kawa River Model: An alternative occupational perspective. Poster presented at the 20th-23rd June 2006 College of Occupational Therapy Annual Conference, Cardiff.

Lim KH (2006b) Applying the Kawa Model. In: M Iwama (ed.) *The Kawa River Model: Culturally Relevant Occupational Therapy*. Edinburgh: Elsevier Churchill Livingstone.

Lim KH, Iwama M (2006) Emerging models – an Asian perspective: The Kawa River Model. In: E Duncan (ed.) *Hagedorn's Foundations for Practice in Occupational Therapy*. Edinburgh: Elsevier Churchill Livingstone.

Macpherson W (1999) *The Macpherson Report*. HMSO Command Paper No. 4262-I London: HMSO.

Masi R (1992) Communication: cross-cultural applications of the physician's art. *Canadian Family Physician, 38(May)*, 1159–1165.

McGruder J (2003) Culture, race, ethnicity and human diversity. In: EB Crepeau, ES Cohn, BAB Schell (eds). *Willard and Spackman's Occupational Therapy*. (10th edn) Baltimore, MD: Lippincott Williams and Wilkins.

Mind (2002) *Statistics on Race, Culture and Mental Health*. London: Mind Publications.

Mintzberg H (1983) *Power In and Around Organizations*. Englewood Cliffs, NJ: Prentice-Hall.

Office for National Statistics (2001) *National Census 2001*, London: HMSO.

Office for National Statistics (2005) *Immigrant Statistics*, London: HMSO.

Office of Deputy Prime Minister (2004) *Social Exclusion and Mental Health Report*. London: HMSO.

Reynolds F, Lim KH (2005) The social context of older people. In: A McIntyre, A Atwal (eds) *Occupational Therapy and Older People*. Oxford: Blackwell Publishing, 27–48.

Sainsbury Centre for Mental Health (2000) *Breaking the Circle of Fear*. London: Sainsbury Centre for Mental Health Publication.

Sainsbury Centre for Mental Health (2002) *Breaking the Circle of Fear: A Review of the Relationship between Mental Health Services and African and Caribbean Communities*. London: Sainsbury Centre for Mental Health Publication.

Secker J, Harding C (2002) African and African Caribbean user's perceptions of inpatient services. *Journal of Psychiatric and Mental Health Nursing*, 9(2), 161–168.

Servan-Schreiber D (2004) *Healing without Freud or Prozac*. London: Rodale.

Smith HC (2005) 'Feel the FEAR AND DO IT ANYWAY': Meeting the Occupational Needs of refugees and People Seeking Asylum. *British Journal of Occupational Therapy, 68(10)*, 474–476.

Sortland G (2006) A content analysis of current mental health policy in reference to mental health promotion and minority ethnic communities. Brunel University: Unpublished MSc dissertation.

Townsend E (1999) Enabling occupation in the 21st century: making good intentions a reality. *Australian Occupational Therapy Journal, 46(4)*, 147–159.

Tribe P (2002) Mental health of refugees and asylum seekers. *Advances in Psychiatric treatments, 4(3)*, 1–8.

Trivedi P(1999) Unanswered questions: A user's perspective. In: K Bhui, D Olajide (eds) *Mental Health Service Provision: For a Multi-Cultural Society*. London: Saunders, 11–20.

Trivedi, P (2002) Racism, Social Exclusion and Mental Health: A Black User's Perspective. In: K Bhui (ed.) *Racism and Mental Health*. London: Jessica Kingsley, 71–82.

Wells SA, Black RM (2000) *Cultural Competency for Health Professionals*. New York: The American Occupational Therapy Association, Inc.

Wetherell M (1996) Group conflict and the social psychology of racism. In: M Wetherell (ed.) *Identities, Groups and Social Issues*. London: Sage, 175–238.

Whiteford G (2000) Occupational deprivation: global challenge in the new millennium. *British Journal of Occupational Therapy*, 63(5), 200–204.

Wilcock AA (2006) *An Occupational Perspective of Health*. Thorofare, NJ: Slack.

Wilson M, Francis J (1997) *Raised Voices*. London: Mind Publications

World Federation of Occupational Therapists (2006) *Position Statement on Human Rights*. Victoria, Australia: WFOT, 1–2.

Part II Exploring Practice Contexts

4 Engaging the disengaged
Practising in acute in-patient settings

Samantha Dewis and Michelle Harrison

Personal narrative

For many occupational therapists, on graduating and wanting to work within mental health services, we find ourselves working within a hospital-based, acute in-patient unit – a place where we plan to develop our skills, learn the tools of our trade and finally put into practice the knowledge and skills we have learned so far. But identifying and defining these skills is challenging, as is deciding whether a special set of skills is required to work in acute mental health settings.

With the international move towards community-based mental health services, the past decade has seen a wealth of opportunities emerge for occupational therapists working within traditional and non-traditional community mental heath settings. However, the development of these services has adversely influenced the quality of in-patient mental health services. In the UK, this inequality of provision has been acknowledged, with a consequent increase in funding for in-patient services (Lim *et al.*, 2007). Despite this high investment in in-patient services, they are still often perceived as a last resort, with consistent low levels of service user satisfaction and significant problems recruiting and retaining staff. As the focus of mental health services has changed to keep people out of hospital and supported within their own homes by community-based services, the population of mental health in-patient units has changed significantly with shorter lengths of stay.

In the UK, acute mental health units have become an increasingly challenging environment for staff and service users alike. Patients admitted to wards are at their most distressed and vulnerable, the likelihood being that community services have been unable to offer the support necessary or that individuals have required compulsory admission under the Mental Health Act (1983). The Sainsbury Centre for Mental Health (SCMH) (1998) in their report on acute services notes that it is at this time of vulnerability that people are in most in need of good-quality sensitive care.

Having worked within acute mental health for the majority of our professional careers so far, we feel strongly that the work of occupational therapists within acute in-patient settings needs greater acknowledgement, reflection and debate. There is very little published material guiding the work of occupational therapists in this setting; yet for many occupational therapists, this is their first post-qualifying experience. The published work highlights the negative and often risk-laden experiences of service users and staff on acute admission wards. With the changing needs of the in-patient population and the seemingly increasing use of the Mental Health Act to detain individuals, there is an inevitable impact upon our work. We must therefore ask ourselves whether there is still a valid, safe and relevant role for occupational therapy. We believe that there most definitely is; however, our concern is how we support this within an evidence-based framework. So, this is why there is a need to write about the work of occupational therapy in this setting.

This chapter will challenge the reader to explore the scope of occupational therapy within an acute mental health setting and consider the knowledge and skills we need to engage people experiencing an acute episode of mental ill health. We will use a case study to reflect on how our core skills can be used to effectively and confidently to engage individuals in the occupational therapy process. We will also consider how we can begin to overcome the barriers faced on a daily basis within acute mental health units and how we can be part of a multi-disciplinary, therapeutic approach to in-patient care.

Case Study 4.1 John's story

John, a 45-year-old man, was admitted to an acute admission ward following a relapse in his mental state. He has a long history of schizophrenia and chronic negative symptoms, poor motivation, social withdrawal and blunted mood. On admission he was paranoid, aggressive and responding to voices. John has a history of non-compliance with medication and poor self-care. Prior to admission he was living in a supported housing project and was known to the assertive outreach team. He did not attend any day services within the community. During the multi-disciplinary ward review, it was decided to refer him to occupational therapy to assess his living skills. John is currently spending his time on the ward in his room, lying on the settee in the television room or smoking cigarettes.

Acute admission wards

John is a familiar case example for occupational therapists working on acute admission wards. With minimal information and a broad reason for referral, the expectation from the referrer is that the occupational therapist will carry out a thorough assessment of John's living skills. According to Creek (2003), the occupational therapy process now begins. There is now a reason for referral and need for the occupational therapist to begin to gather information from a number of different sources.

As John has been known to mental health services for some years, a wealth of information was available about him, including data gathered from his current admission, contact with the assertive outreach service, his care plan prior to admission to hospital and his most recent risk assessment. However, working with John in a collaborative, meaningful and mutually agreed-upon occupational therapy assessment and intervention process is yet to begin.

Engaging the patient

There is little written about how to engage individuals in the occupational therapy process within acute mental health settings. However, the need for this process to occur is acknowledged by Creek (2003) in her work defining occupational therapy as a complex intervention. In this she recognises that the occupational therapist must work 'assertively to engage people in need who are considered likely to benefit from intervention' (p. 20). In this context, there may be need for a pre-assessment stage, a precursor to formal intervention, whereby the core skills of the occupational therapist are used to prior to the formal assessment process.

Creek (2003, p.18) goes on to propose that, for the experienced practitioner, the occupational therapy process is often not the linear one first perceived. Instead, the occupational therapist's skills and knowledge are translated into 'action targeted at particular groups of people', which, in this context, are people who are acutely mentally ill, such as John, admitted to mental health admission wards.

The process of involving people in this pre-assessment, information-gathering stage, using activities that are meaningful and therapeutic to them is lengthy and intensive and requires constant revisiting. Spending time just being with an individual can help lay the foundations for a therapeutic relationship. Both the patient and the occupational therapist should understand the value of how and why the time taken in engagement is an important part of intervention.

The challenge and skill required to actively engage people during an acute episode of mental ill health can be a source of great frustration for practitioners. Chadwick and Birchwood (1996) suggest that the factors that may prevent engagement with those experiencing such serious mental illness include the inability of mental health staff to empathise with the patients' experience of symptoms because they are outside the realm of the staff's own experience. Engagement is not the sole responsibility of any one profession; instead, it is a common, shared multi-disciplinary skill that must be valued by all involved. Star Wards (2006, p. 5) is a document that describes the value of increasing patient engagement on acute wards. 'Service users want it, staff want it. Managers want it. Carers, commissioners, councillors. Everyone believes that time spent on acute wards should be actively therapeutic and patients should have the option of a constructive programme of activities each day.'

Clinical reasoning

It is important that professionals take responsibility for their reasoning skills and ability to reflect on how these skills are used creatively in working with individuals.

Here, the problem-solving process, a core concept and value within occupational therapy, can be helpful. Robertson (1996) describes how a problem can arise when someone wants to do something – in this case, to engage John in the occupational therapy process of assessment and intervention – but does not know how to or is blocked in some way from employing a previously used solution – in this example, a formal assessment of John's living skills.

The ability of occupational therapists to problem solve and critically analyse clinical decision-making processes develops with experience. In her work observing the therapist with the 'three track mind' Fleming (1991) noted that occupational therapists use different modes of clinical reasoning and thinking in different situations, according to the problem identified. She observed that experienced occupational therapists were able to move smoothly from one mode of thinking to another, guiding the reasoning process through multiple, diverse problems faced by the patient. In the clinical decision-making process with John, the complexities of Fleming's three strands can be clearly identified. As with the occupational therapy process, three-strand reasoning is not linear; instead, the work of engaging John is complicated and must be carried out beyond his specific problems and within the wider context of his admission to hospital. Fleming (1991, p. 1012) observed that 'this thinking process is essentially imagination tempered by clinical experience and expertise'.

McKay (1999) specifically discusses clinical reasoning in an acute mental health setting. She describes how the occupational therapist, Lillian, and the patient, Paula, worked together in an acute ward. The range and complexity of information gleaned throughout an individual's hospital stay requires the therapist to utilise a range of reasoning processes to make sense of the client's life and then to use various ways of working to engage and sustain involvement with the client. McKay proposed a clinical reasoning model in acute mental health setting, which is informed and constructed by four key components: the working environment, the client, the therapeutic context and the therapist. These aspects can be examined separately, but they all need to be considered to enable the therapist to construct an image of the client and their resultant therapeutic response (McKay, 1999).

See Case Study 4.1

John has begun to talk more readily for brief periods of time with nursing and occupational therapy staff and is able to request that his basic needs be met. When asked why he stays in his room for most of the day, or can be found watching television, John states that there is nothing else to do.

Returning to the case study, as John considers that there is nothing to do other than stay in bed or watch television, the occupational therapist is challenged to motivate his participation in activities that are meaningful to him when faced with such negative symptoms and lack of motivation. The observation that his basic needs are being met may be considered through the work of Maslow (1954) who first proposed a hierarchy of human needs that culminate in self-actualisation. Maslow believed that humans are subject to two levels of motivational force – those that ensure survival by satisfying basic physical and psychological needs and those that promote self-actualisation. Maslow goes on to emphasise that the needs lower in the hierarchy must be satisfied before the higher needs can be considered.

Applying Maslow's theory to the services available to patients in acute admission wards, it can be conceptualised the basic needs of food, warmth and shelter are provided although there is some doubt about safety, another of the other basic needs, with some literature highlighting acute wards as unsafe environments [SCMH, 1998; Royal College of Psychiatrists (RCP), 2005]. However, the environment is unlikely to empower patients to strive toward self-actualisation during their admission.

Roberts (1997) considered the need to empower individuals experiencing mental ill health. Using the work of Maslow, he acknowledged the close links between self-actualisation, creativity and empowerment and the role of occupational therapists in this process. However, he also encouraged practitioners to reflect upon just how difficult it is to achieve self-actualisation: 'It's no good telling clients to be more creative, we cannot make others creative, nor can we let it happen. But occupational therapy is about helping clients take this power on themselves' (Roberts, 1997, p. 15).

Meaningful occupation or boredom?

As will be illustrated, whilst much published work refers to the importance of involving patients in recreation or therapeutic groups during their stay on acute admission wards, there is very little specific acknowledgement to meaningful occupation within this context. Although the concept of meaningful occupation is familiar to occupational therapists, other professions struggle to make sense of it. Instead, the term boredom is often used by service users and other professions, a concept that many occupational therapists struggle with and feel threatened by. Rebeiro (1998) considered occupation to be a basic human need, directly related to the meaning and quality of life. If occupational therapists could translate boredom as simply being a lack of occupation and thus a lack of meaning and quality to life, it becomes a much more palatable translation for a commonly used but misunderstood word.

Binnema (2004) considered boredom to be an emotion linked to meaning; therefore, to address many of the difficulties faced by service users in mental health wards, the consequences of boredom must be considered. Boredom is the word consistently used to describe what patients experience in acute mental health wards in the UK. The SCMH (1998) describes how patients receive only limited therapeutic input and are subsequently bored during their stay in hospital. The Royal College of Psychiatrists' (2005) national audit of violence on mental health wards identifies high levels of boredom as a factor contributing to unsafe wards.

The Department of Health (2001), in its guidelines for adult acute in-patient care in the UK, recommends a high level of therapeutic interventions and an interactive environment to diminish the levels of disturbances, violence and boredom.

Whilst few documents go on to offer practical solutions to this problem, one recent publication does. Written with service user involvement at its core, Star Wards (2006) offers practical and simple ways for improving the experiences and treatment outcomes of acute mental health in-patients. The paper begins to recognise the benefit and functional qualities of, in particular, recreational activities beyond just dealing with boredom.

Occupational therapists working within the acute mental health setting must begin to tackle what boredom really means. Polemeni-Walker et al. (1992) explored the reasons why individuals attended occupational therapy within an in-patient setting. They went on to express their concerns whether patients were gaining the optimal benefits from attending therapeutic groups when patients viewed the relief of boredom as the most important reason for participating.

Defining groups and the role of occupational therapists in facilitating these is important. Harries and Caan (1994) asked both patients and ward staff what they thought of occupational therapy. A common perception was that occupational therapy had a role in providing relief from boredom. In response to this, Harries and Cann (1994) suggested that 'rather than trying to become entertainers, occupational therapists might try to meet the need by developing the patients' skills to entertain themselves'. The misconception about the role of occupational therapists continues to be an issue more that a decade later. When Simpson et al. (2005) carried out their study of multi-disciplinary working on an acute mental health ward, they believed that there continued to be the misperception that occupational therapists were there to keep people busy and prevent idleness.

The process of encouraging people to participate in occupations meaningful to them means considering the value of doing and the value of activity. Finlay (2004) describes the centrality of occupation and the healing power of activity with both the process and the final product having an intrinsic value. Nagle et al. (2002) explored the relationship between individuals' state of health and occupational performance and, while this study was based in a community mental health vocational setting, there are relevant comparisons with the experiences of people admitted to acute mental health wards. They noted that individuals have rich and diverse occupational histories that are part of their current identities and that influence their occupational choice. However, they also reported that the individuals themselves recognised the risk of exacerbating their symptoms by attempting to do too much or being overstimulated. This has implications for the nature of an acute admission ward and emphasises the importance of having an environment that facilitates engagement without overstimulating individuals.

Whilst John currently experiences negative symptoms and poor motivation that limit his participation, it is essential to explore activities that would encourage and motivate him. He is, without doubt, occupationally deprived and disadvantaged. Wilcock (1999) regards the consequences of occupational deprivation as people being unable play a full part in the world around them through diminished interactions.

Occupational deprivation then leaves people less able to make sense of their world or themselves, an all-too-familiar occurrence on acute mental health wards.

The result of John's lack of meaningful occupation, both prior to admission and on the ward, can lead to a number of unresolved stressors and occupational risk factors. Fieldhouse (2000) suggests such unresolved stressors ultimately manifest themselves in states such as boredom, burnout and sleep disturbance. If, during John's in-patient admission, the multi-disciplinary team do not attempt to involve or engage him in any meaningful activity, it could be argued that they are, in fact, extending his occupational alienation and deprivation.

The responsibility of engaging John is a multi-disciplinary process in its initial stages. Occupational therapists in these teams can use their knowledge and skills to guide and support nursing staff in continuing to engage with John throughout his day, using recreational and social activities to do so. Activities do not have to be complicated or expensive; the occupational therapist needs to be creative with ideas and resources. A pack of cards, a newspaper or a magazine can provide a wealth of information and interaction. The Internet holds host to an infinite number of free resources, whether accessed directly or downloaded for use. Therapists should not be afraid to be creative and resourceful or to do ordinary things. Activities that are often taken for granted or accessible within an individual's home are often limited, under-resourced or simply unavailable in an acute mental health ward.

Taking the time to engage with John in activities he enjoys, such as watching television or reading a newspaper, and being consistent in this approach will allow the occupational therapist to begin the process of assessment and intervention with John. Engagement requires both professional and personal skills; anecdotal evidence from both authors of this chapter suggests that conversations that take place over a game of cards or a newspaper crossword can be powerful and memorable for both the service user and the professional, building the trust and knowledge from which further assessment and intervention takes place. There is no instruction manual on how to do this, and it takes confidence, knowledge and skill on the part of the professional. Perhaps most importantly, it breaks down barriers and challenges misconceptions that professionals have about themselves and service users.

Activity analysis is important. By breaking down and analysing an activity, such as reading and discussing a newspaper article, a number of different skills are used, such as concentration, orientation, communication and interaction. This core skill is invaluable for working within this setting.

See Case Study 4.1

During a conversation with John one day, he discloses his dislike of the breakfast provided on the ward. He goes on to describe his past enjoyment of cooking a breakfast each weekend as a Sunday morning treat.

Occupational engagement

Finlay (2004) discusses the challenges in engaging individuals in activity. She describes the process that occupational therapists follow as they seek to interest people and motivate them to be active when their impulse is to do the reverse. In doing this, she argues, that account must be taken of the special meaning particular occupations have for that individual.

In their study of the relationship between an individual's state of health and their occupational performance, Nagle *et al.* (2002) note that although people will resume occupational engagement when they feel better, their illness will continue to influence and alter their occupational choices. To maintain their mental health, individuals sought out daily occupations that had structure, flexibility and demands that could be easily met, thus giving them control over their actions. Routine and structure was also reported by Chugg and Craik (2002) as factors influencing the occupational engagement of people with schizophrenia living in the community. Such factors can be as relevant to people admitted to hospital. Identifying what is important for people prior to their admission assists the process of involving them in relevant and meaningful occupation and occupational therapy intervention whilst they are in-patients.

Charmaz (2002) addressed the experiences of people with chronic illnesses and the challenges faced in gaining concordance. Again, many of the issues can be translated to working with people with chronic mental health problems, such as John. She acknowledged the difficulties faced with compliance when patient and practitioner hold divergent opinions about the condition and intervention, particularly if these involve a change to the daily habits of the patient. Concordance can only resume when both patient and practitioner have a shared understanding of the individual's needs and situation and agree on the benefits of the intervention.

In their study of the views of 64 in-patients of occupational therapy in a large London mental health service, Lim *et al.* (2007) reported that group intervention with an occupational focus that patients judged to be meaningful and relevant was most beneficial. Sporting activities and cookery were reported as the most beneficial activities. There was a highly significant and positive correlation between occupational therapy meeting the needs of individuals and improving their daily functioning and quality of their admission. However, in-patients would have preferred to be more involved in deciding on their individual goals and targets. This emphasis on cookery echoes the finding of Haley and McKay (2004), also in an acute mental health setting, where patients' views of baking were elicited by semi-structured interview. They appreciated the productive aspect of baking, which had meaning for them and they could appreciate the befefits of their participation.

Despite John's long history of admissions to hospital and contact with mental health services, it is essential that his understanding and beliefs about his diagnosis and, more specifically, subsequent difficulties in engaging with meaningful occupations are established. It is only then that the process of understanding and sharing John's future occupational needs can begin.

The occupational therapist must recognise the cues revealed during the invaluable time spent just talking, without a more formal assessment process taking place. Through this an understanding of an individual's roles, routines and habits can be gained. In conversation, John expressed a dislike of the food available to him in hospital and recalled a past enjoyment of his Sunday treat, an occupation that had special meaning to him. Finlay (2004) describes the intrinsic and extrinsic value of activity and the importance of how an activity is applied to the individual. John has provided a gateway into engaging him in assessment and intervention. He can now be brought into a more familiar occupational therapy process, using the cues given about his past enjoyment of cooking breakfast to participate in more formal assessments and interventions.

> **See Case Study 4.1**
>
> John agrees to use the occupational therapy department kitchen to cook a bacon sandwich for his breakfast. During the time spent in the kitchen with the occupational therapist, he begins to engage in the assessment process and is willing to consider attending further occupational therapy sessions available to him. The occupational therapist is able to begin the occupational therapy process of assessment and intervention.

This example of using the overtly simple activity of cooking as a gateway to stimulate interest in other occupations is reflected in the studies by Haley and McKay (2004) and Lim *et al.* (2007). The occupation has wide relevance and acceptability and had meanings at different levels for different people at different times.

Summary

The value of taking time to really listen to John and engage him in his story and narrative is the key to involving him in occupations that are relevant and meaningful in his journey through mental health recovery. Smith (2006) observed that it is people's stories that allow therapists to make the connection between them and their practice. For many patients, having the opportunity to tell their story can often start during an in-patient admission. It can also continue episodically as individuals find themselves re-admitted to hospital during other stages in their life. In the present authors' experiences, stories are told when people relax, when they are engrossed in a game of dominoes or when they are chatting over a cup of tea or reading a newspaper. By taking the time to listen to people telling their story, we can begin to encourage their participation in activities that have meaning and relevance to them, and as time progresses, a therapeutic relationship develops before the more formal process of assessment and intervention.

The chapter has begun to address the complexity, yet also the simplicity, in engaging the disengaged. To occupational therapists what appears to others as a simple conversation over a game of dominoes involves a complex series of clinical reasoning and activity analysis processes and skills to engage the disengaged individual. As practitioners we must be clear about what our intervention entails at every level, both for the understanding of the service user, ourselves and our multi-disciplinary colleagues. We must also understand the complexity of needs of people admitted to acute mental health admission wards, never underestimating the nature and risk involved when individuals are acutely and floridly unwell.

The problems facing staff working within acute mental health settings are widely acknowledged and the media are quick to highlight dangers and inadequacies. Wards are often under-resourced and boredom is undoubtedly a huge problem for in-patients. However, there is much excellent work carried out and we must be confident to highlight this: 'Staff and patients need to have scope to let their aptitudes and skills flourish, working together in partnership and promoting self management' (Star Wards, 2006, p. 4).

As occupational therapists working within acute in-patient settings, we have a key role to play in supporting individuals to reconnect with their lives through activities that have meaning to them. Often these are daily activities, which we take for granted and are easily accessible to us in a non-ward environment. However, in a ward, these activities are inaccessible, and ultimately, individuals are disempowered and disengaged. As a profession we must be proud of our core skills and our expertise about what we can discover through the medium of activity and creative use of resources. We must also be confident to go ahead and establish and evidence base for our work.

Questioning your Practice

1. How can occupational therapy support individuals who are occupationally disempowered to regain, maintain and develop meaningful occupation during admission to hospital?
2. Consider the resources available to you; are you using them flexibly and creatively to meet the needs of the in-patient population?
3. How do we prove the effectiveness of occupational therapy to ensure service users and their carers benefit from occupation specific interventions during admission to acute mental health in-patient units?

References

Binnema D (2004) Inter relations of psychiatric patient experiences of boredom and mental health. *Issues in Mental Health Nursing, (25)*, 833–842.

Chadwick P, Birchwood M (1996) *Cognitive Therapy for Delusions, Voices and Paranoia*. Chichester: John Wiley & Sons.

Charmaz C (2002) The self as habit: The reconstruction of self in chronic illness. *Occupational Therapy Journal of Rehabilitation, (22)*, 31s–41s.

Chugg A, Craik C (2002) Some factors influencing occupational engagement for people with schizophrenia living in the community. *British Journal of Occupational Therapy, 65(2),* 67–73.

Creek J (2003) *Defining Occupational Therapy as a Complex Intervention.* London: College of Occupational Therapists.

Department of Health (1983) *The Mental Health Act.* London: HMSO.

Department of Health (2001) *The Mental Health Policy Implementation Guide.* London: Department of Health.

Fieldhouse J (2000) Occupational science and community mental health: using occupational risk factors as a framework for exploring chronicity. *British Journal of Occupational Therapy, 63(5),* 211–217.

Finlay L (2004) *The Practice of Psychosocial Occupational Therapy.* (3rd edn) London: Nelson Thornes.

Fleming MH (1991) The therapist with the three-track mind. *The American Journal of Occupational Therapy, 45(11),* 1007–1014.

Haley L, McKay EA (2004) 'Baking gives you confidence': users' views of engaging in the occupation of baking. *British Journal of Occupational Therapy, 67(3),* 125–128.

Harries P, Caan AW (1994) What do psychiatric inpatients and ward staff think about occupational therapy? *British Journal of Occupational Therapy, 57(6),* 219–223.

Lim KH, Morris J, Craik C (2007) Inpatients' perspectives of occupational therapy in acute mental health. *Australian Occupational Therapy Journal, 54(4),* 22 –32.

Maslow A (1954) *Motivation and Personality.* New York: Harper & Row.

McKay EA (1999) Lillian and Paula: A treatment narrative in acute mental health. In: SE Ryan, EA McKay (eds) *Thinking and Reasoning in Therapy,* 53–64. Cheltenham: Stanley Thornes, 53–64.

Nagle S, Valient C, Polatajko H (2002) I'm doing as much as I can: occupational choices persons with a severe and persistent mental illness. *Journal of Occupational Science, 9(2),* 72–81.

Polimeni-Walker I, Wilson KG, Jewers R (1992) Reasons for participating in occupational therapy groups: perceptions of adult psychiatric inpatients and occupational therapists. *Canadian Journal of Occupational Therapy, 59(5),* 240–247.

Rebeiro KL (1998) Occupation-as-means to mental health: a review of the literature, and a call for research. *Canadian Journal of Occupational Therapy, 65(1),* 12–19.

Roberts G (1997) Mental health occupational therapy: action, creativity and service. *Mental Health Occupational Therapy, 2(1),* 10–16.

Robertson LJ (1996) Clinical reasoning, Part 1: the nature of problem solving, a literature review. *British Journal of Occupational Therapy, 59(4),* 178–182.

Royal College of Psychiatrists (2005) *National Audit of Violence 2003-2005 Final Report.* London: Royal College of Psychiatrists Research Unit.

Sainsbury Centre for Mental Health (1998) *Acute Problems: A Survey of the Quality of Care in Acute Psychiatric Wards.* London: Sainsbury Centre for Mental health.

Simpson A, Bowers L, Alexander J, Ridley C and Warren J (2005) Occupational therapy and multidisciplinary working on acute psychiatric wards: the Tompkins acute ward study. *British Journal of Occupational Therapy, 68(12),* 545-552.

Smith G (2006) The Casson memorial lecture 2006: telling tales – how stories and narrative co-create change. *British Journal of Occupational Therapy, 69(7),* 304–311.

Star Wards (2006) Practical ideas for improving the daily experiences and treatment outcomes of acute mental health in-patients. http://brightplace.org.uk/pdfs/starwards.pdf Accessed 14th Feb. 2007.

Wilcock AA (1999) Reflections on doing, being and becoming. *Australian Occupational Therapy Journal, 4,* 1–11.

5 Broadening horizons
Beyond acute mental health

Michelle Harrison and Samantha Dewis

Personal narratives

As occupational therapists, we both have been involved in acute mental health practice for the majority of our professional careers. Our journeys have been very different, but we have arrived at a similar point in terms of what we feel is important for occupational therapy as a profession and in practice. We both feel strongly about the integral part activity and occupation play as therapy in mental health practice and how this is defined by the service user and the therapist. We also have extensive experience of involving service users as colleagues in programme delivery and service evaluation. This experience has greatly influenced our practice and the way we have subsequently designed and delivered services.

As mental health services have rapidly developed in the UK to meet the needs of service users in their homes and communities, we have observed that occupational therapists are not always evident in emerging areas of practice even though there is a clear need for their skills. These observations are not unique to the UK and have been reported internationally where similar restructuring of mental health services has occurred.

Personal experience has led us to conclude that working with service users in the most acute stages of their illness requires advanced practice skills, whether this is in a hospital environment or in crisis/home treatment teams. Traditionally, working in hospitals has been regarded as the safe option because of the inherent environmental structure provided. However, occupational therapy has been challenged to meet the needs of people in the acute stages of their illness, whether they are admitted to hospital or cared for in the community. We both feel that, as part of our involvement in this changing environment, we need to recognise the work that occupational therapists can offer to service users at this time in their recovery journey.

Introduction

There has been ongoing debate in the occupational therapy literature about whether occupational therapists are best placed to work with service users in crisis outside the confines of hospital (Rosenfield,1984; Miller & Robertson,1991). In the UK, policy has recommended a change of focus away from treating the majority of clients in crisis in the hospital environment to alternative settings and home treatment (Department of Health, 2001). Policy in the US, Australia and Canada has also taken this direction (Polak & Kirby, 1976; Miller & Robertson,1991; Gage,1995; Lloyd *et al.*, 1999). There are multiple reasons for this change in the management of service users. Some of this has been as a response to service users' preference for alternative treatment options, allowing them a greater input into what happens when they experience a crisis. Another key consideration is finance, enabling money previously spent on in-patient bed days to be redirected and used more cost-effectively in alternative community service provision. Socially, interventions provided in the community allow for greater involvement of the people important to the service user, whether these are friends, family members or health care professionals.

Although the benefits of these changes are recognised by occupational therapists, there is ongoing deliberation within the profession regarding generic versus specialist roles, especially when working in the community (Parker, 2001; Cook, 2003; Harries & Gilhooly, 2003; Harrison, 2003). A search of the occupational therapy literature demonstrates that there is no discussion of this area of practice in relation to in-patient and community crisis work, and what these emerging roles may look like or how therapists would experience these.

It is often considered that crisis intervention posts involve non-traditional or extended scope practice, which are frequently considered as generic. Take-up of these posts is not only a choice for the profession as a whole but also for the individual practitioner. However, there are specialist skills associated with these roles, and occupational therapists need to acknowledge that they may have developed these skills as part of their existing clinical experience and can transfer them into these alternative settings and situations.

In all areas of occupational therapy it is likely that practitioners will encounter service users at a stage of crisis or when they have to adjust to the impact of crisis on their occupational performance. This may be a traumatic injury, a loss or a relapse of illness; whatever the cause, when considering a person in crisis, the occupational therapist reflects on how a crisis impacts them as individuals and their occupational functioning in their environment. Working with service users in an acute mental health crisis is no different, and employs the same skills. It is acknowledged that most crises for service users in mental health are a result of social or emotional stressors. Therefore, the management of a crisis is not necessarily defined by symptoms that require a medical approach to deal with them. The person in crisis may find ways to resolve his or her problems or may find it increasingly difficult to deal with the situation that causes further disruption to his or her daily life, the things that are important to him or her and his or her ability to maintain their usual routines. The ability to assess the service users' needs at the point of crisis, working alongside them to resolve the crisis and ensuring their return to health, are familiar to most occupational therapists.

Crisis

Caplan (1964) is widely cited in the literature for his early recognition and definition of a crisis. He described four phases of a crisis:

- Phase 1 – Tension mounting.
- Phase 2 – Increasing disorganisation.
- Phase 3 – Mobilisation of all internal and external resources.
- Phase 4 – Major disorganisation or maladaption.

Later, Onyett (1998, p. 156) further elaborated these phases as follows:

1. The individual is confronted by a problem that poses a threat to perceived needs, and habitual problem-solving strategies are used in response.
2. If these familiar strategies fail, feelings of stress escalate and encourage trial and error attempts at problem solving. These will normally be new to the individual and it is at this point that crises offer potential for new learning.
3. If the trial-and-error attempts are not successful, ineffective emergency measures may be attempted to alleviate the problem.
4. If these fail, stress increases to a level beyond the individual's capacity to cope, and psychological dysfunction ensues to such a degree that the user may need to leave or be removed from the situation.

These descriptions will be familiar to occupational therapists, especially those working in acute in-patient units, who are likely to have encountered service users at both stages three and four of a crisis. The Mental Health Foundation (2003) asked service users how hospitals helped at times of crisis, what coping strategies were used to reduce mental distress and what could the hospital do better to help them cope. Service users reported that activities that motivated them were helpful but that 'the need for sanctuary during times of crisis is jeopardised by the poor relationship between staff and patients' (p. 3). Significantly, they also identified that service users were not being provided with appropriate and timely support at times of crisis. Lelliot and Quirk (2004), in reviewing the literature on acute hospital admissions from several countries, highlighted that one group of inpatients in Norway had identified their common needs on admission as being 'security, sleep, rest and help with finding meaning, which includes "new tracks in life" and an ability to cope better with difficult situations' (p. 299). Both these studies emphasised the need for timely support in an environment to sustain the service user in crisis, whether it is an in-patient unit or at home. With the introduction of crisis resolution/home treatment teams, there has gradually been a change in the needs of the service users admitted to in-patient units, resulting in more intensive input from all staff members in the unit. Importantly, there has also been a general reduction in length of stay for service users, which decreases the likelihood of dependency but may leave individuals feeling insecure and unsupported in the community.

Crisis intervention teams

Crisis intervention teams were established to 'prevent where possible, hospitalisation, deterioration of symptoms and stress experienced by relatives/others involved in the crisis situation' (Hopkins and Wasley, 2002, p. 18). Birchwood *et al.* (1998) discussed the value of working with service users to identify their relapse signatures, identifying their early warning signs and using them to prevent, where possible, complete relapse and admission to hospital.

Dealing with crisis in the home environment is usually seen as preferable for service users. However, a study on referral patterns to crisis resolution teams followed up service users subsequently admitted to hospitals. It demonstrated that there remained a group of service users who chose to be admitted to hospital rather than to receive treatment at home (Brimblecombe, 2000). This aspect was not investigated further in the study, but it may be that these service users only feel safe away from their home environment at such times of crisis. As hospital admission has been the usual response for service users in crisis, a change in approach may take some time to be accepted by service users and staff alike.

In-patient units

The state of in-patient mental health units and the service they provide in England has been widely criticised [The Sainsbury Centre for Mental Health (SCMH), 1998; Ford, 1999; Campbell, 2000; Dratcu, 2002]. Recent reviews of in-patient care report only limited improvement of facilities and services available to service users. Occupational therapists, in a study by Simpson *et al.* (2005), expressed their frustration at service users either being too ill to engage in activities or being discharged just as they are engaging fully in therapeutic activities. Similarly, nursing staff often feel that the emphasis of nursing care is directed towards the 'management of dangerous behaviours and patient throughput' (Lelliot & Quirk, 2004, p. 300). They are also dissatisfied about the lack of time to engage with service users beyond the immediate pressures that present themselves. Duffy and Nolan (2005) and Simpson *et al.* (2005) reported that occupational therapists working in acute hospital environments were discouraged by the multi-disciplinary teams' misunderstanding of their role. These frustrations may have contributed to an 'exodus' of staff from acute wards to new community teams, such as assertive outreach and crisis teams, as reported by Dennis-Jones (2005).

Transition to crisis intervention

For occupational therapists, the move away from traditional hospital departments to community outreach and in-reach programmes and other new ways of working such as in crisis resolution teams is challenging. Gage (1995) in Canada and

Lloyd *et al.* (1999) in Australia found that occupational therapists faced similar issues when ways of working changed. These changes are often perceived as a threat. There appears to be two areas of concern: the move away from working within an occupational therapy team and having to use additional skills in conjunction with core expertise.

Perhaps, there is an inherent safety net in working within a team of occupational therapists in an in-patient unit where there is a readily available pool of colleagues who can offer informal support and understand the struggles that the practitioner faces. However, the frustration of working in the hospital is that environmental factors affect the occupational therapist's ability to carry out intervention. For example, lack of physical space and resources, the diverse needs of service users admitted to in-patient units, unpredictable ward environments and policy and procedures restrict the ability to carry out interventions. The frustrations of in-patient work can affect both the occupational therapists' satisfaction with their work with service users and the service users' experience of occupational therapy during admission.

Conversely, working in crisis resolution can offer the occupational therapist the opportunity to work with service users in their own environment, using the service users' own resources such as familiar objects and people. However, each crisis team is likely to have only one occupational therapist; so support from other occupational therapy colleagues can be limited. Finding allies in a team who will provide support is invaluable. But regular professional supervision by an occupational therapist allows practitioners to retain their occupational therapy focus while reflecting on their experience of working in different ways that incorporate some generic team tasks. This supervision is also an important aspect of continuing professional development.

Case Study 5.1   Alison's story

Following an initial assessment Alison, 35, was referred to the occupational therapist working within a crisis intervention team. The reason for the specific referral to occupational therapy was to support Alison in maintaining her role and activities of daily living during this period of crisis in an attempt to prevent admission to hospital.

Prior to this particular crisis, Alison had been working 20 hours a week as a nursing assistant in her local GP surgery, where she has worked for the past 10 years. Alison lives with her husband of 12 years and two children aged 8 and 6.

Alison has experienced one previous episode of mental ill health, which resulted in admission to hospital and detention under the Mental Health Act (1983). During this time she was given a diagnosis of bipolar disorder. Alison was 20 years old at this time and studying to be a nurse. After this initial 10-week stay in hospital, Alison has been able to manage her mental health needs successfully with support from her community mental health team, a supportive work environment and her family. Her mood has fluctuated during this time, but she has never required hospital admission or intervention from crisis services.

(Continued)

Case Study 5.1 *Continued*

Prior to this referral to the crisis intervention team, Alison was reported to have been becoming increasingly elated in mood and displaying symptoms of a manic episode. On referral it was found that she had not slept for a number of days, was becoming increasingly grandiose and was struggling to maintain any of her usual roles or routines. Alison expressed some insight into these difficulties and was concerned that it would result in admission to hospital.

Alison's family were concerned that she needed to maintain her usual occupational routines and roles as much as possible, despite currently being off work. This allowed the occupational therapist to engage with Alison and to identify and suggest ways of how particiapte in activities could provide routine and maintain and build on her existing occupational ability and insight into her illness. The initial aim was to increase Alison's tolerance to activity and to establish routine as well as maintain relationships.

Quickly establishing and maintaining a routine for Alison amongst the chaos of her current thoughts enabled her to maintain many of her existing occupations and activities of daily living, such as getting the children ready for school, preparing family meals and maintaining the family home. This gave Alison a sense of purpose during the initial stages of intervention and allowed her to begin to make sense of this time of crisis. It also allowed the occupational therapist to contextualise her engagement in routines and activities with future goals to return to work and achieve a work life balance again.

There is no doubt that preserving specialist skills while working in a more generic or extended scope role is a challenge. Lloyd *et al.* (1999) identified how a lack of a clear professional identity may cause insecurity. The need for occupational therapists to identify their core skills and unique contribution within mental health services has been identified as necessary for some time (Craik *et al.*, 1998; Lloyd *et al.*, 1999; Duffy & Nolan 2005). The emphasis is not only on what occupational therapists' core skills are but also how they engage in the change process and incorporate their skills into new ways of thinking and working (Yau, 1995; Gage, 1995; Pattison, 2006).

It is difficult to establish how many occupational therapists work within in-patient units and crisis intervention teams in the UK. It is recognised that there are several very experienced practitioners working with service users at times of crisis. Identifying the core skills they are using in this area of practice and what additional skills they developed will be considered.

There are several facets of core skills that are transferable for the assessment of service users in crisis both in an in-patient unit and in the community. Creek (2003, p. 36) identified the core skills of occupational therapy as 'collaboration with the client; assessment; enablement; problem solving; using activity as a therapeutic tool; group work and environmental adaptation'. To foster core skills in differing working environments, an occupational therapy model could be used to underpin practice. This can provide an occupationally based language to describe intervention both to service users and to other team members, which keeps the focus of intervention occupationally based (Reeves & Summerfield Mann, 2004;

Bowater & Harrison; 2006). Both the Canadian Model of Occupational Performance (CAOT, 1997) and the Model of Human Occupation (Kielhofner, 2002) provide assessments that can be used to assist with the outcome measurement of intervention. Occupational therapy assessments should be used judiciously and may not always fit either with the service users' needs at a time of crisis or with the limited time available to work with the service user in an in-patient unit. These assessments are an option that can guide intervention. They add value to an intervention with a service user when the occupational therapist has to conduct generic assessment as part of their role. Gage (1995), Harrison *et al.* (2001) and Miller and Robertson (1991) all discuss the additional skills required for working in a crisis intervention team. Miller and Robertson (1991) highlight that the role may involve 'supervising medication, providing support to both the client and their family and maintaining a close watch on the client's progress so that changes can be quickly addressed' (p. 145). They also identified that occupational therapists understand the importance of creativity in problem solving and that this is invaluable when working with service users in crisis.

Risk assessment

Assessment of a service user at the time of crisis needs to incorporate thorough risk assessment, whether the service user is an in-patient or in their home environment. The occupational therapist's contribution lies in working with the multidisciplinary team to identify immediate risks for the service user, potential risks if occupations are neglected and to support risk taking as intervention progresses. If most of the risk is eliminated for the service users during a crisis, they are unlikely to adapt and develop skills to cope with future life incidents. Engagement in occupation, whether routine occupations in the home environment, for example, cooking or cleaning, or in activity-based groups in an in-patient setting, for example, creative or leisure activities, can allow for containment of feelings and mastery of a situation, which can lead to feelings of control. The structure and process of engagement can also facilitate discussion of inner conflicts and troubles, which enable the process of problem solving and can also identify real risks in an informal way rather than through a formal risk assessment process. Two unpublished studies (Harrison, 2003; Harrison & Bahia, 2004) demonstrated that service users expressed how engagement in activity had led them to feel more competent to address issues around structuring their day on their return home and to revisit other activities they had not done for some time. Harrison and Bahia (2004) also found that the opportunity to talk to others and express their ideas was extremely important. These ideas included plans to self-harm, fears regarding their return to home life and life roles, and situations within the unit. This has also been reflected in work carried out by Simpson *et al.* (2005). This process of engagement, whether conducted in the home or an in-patient unit, contributes to continued assessment of the service user and can allow risk to be assessed in a contextual way.

Collaboration with service users

Collaboration with service users at times of crisis can be very challenging for both the therapist and the service user. Duffy and Nolan (2005) identified that the client-centred approach taken by occupational therapists was incongruent with the predominantly medical model followed in in-patient units. Both Lane (2000) and Sumsion (2006) acknowledge that there are challenges to client-centred practice in real-life work settings and that to be client centred we must 'actually be client centred in the talk, actions and structure of everyday practice' (Sumsion, 2000, p. 7). At times of crisis a person's ability to make choices or solve a problem may be impaired. Sumsion (2005) notes that the desire to make decisions declines amongst those with acute and severe illnesses. In addition to this, service users may be compulsorily detained in hospital, and remaining client centred when a decision has to be made about a person's safety towards themselves or others can cause tension for the occupational therapist. Honesty and respect for the service user is essential in this situation; acknowledge that decisions made may not have fully incorporated the service user's wishes. Sumsion (2005) noted that, even though they were not familiar with the term, client-centred practice was important to the participants in the study. Introducing some choice into decision making and intervention with service users at a time of crisis is vital to ensuring their future engagement in services. But, occupational therapists must respect that a service user may not want to prioritise occupational needs.

For occupational therapists working with service users in crisis, an occupational focus is important. But joint working is also integral to the best outcome for the service user. This can incorporate work with professional colleagues, the service user and their family, friends and carers. Listening and supporting carers at times of crisis is essential. The knowledge that friends, family members and other carers possess about the service user, when they have noticed a change in the individual's behaviour, a withdrawal from occupations and normal routines can assist in re-engaging the service user during and after a crisis. Copeland (2001) highlights how effective crisis planning can assist carers, family and friends by giving clear direction on what helps the individual at a time of crisis and can relieve the guilt often felt about whether they have taken the right action.

While working in an acute hospital, the second author was involved in the development of an integrated care pathway five years prior to the introduction of crisis intervention teams in the locality. The aim of the pathway was to clearly define the journey for the service user from admission to discharge. One aspect of this was to remove duplication of questions asked of the service user so that medical, nursing and occupational therapy assessment covered different aspects of the service users' current experience. The doctor completed initial assessment on admission and the nursing staff addressed any immediate issues of risk and safety of the person's property and care for dependants. Then, nursing and occupational therapy staff completed a joint assessment within 3 days of the service user's admission. This process enabled occupational therapists to assess all service users, removing the traditional referral process, thus allowing the occupational therapist the freedom to decide with the service user and their nursing colleagues the importance of occupation and occupational performance at the time of the crisis, while they were on the ward and when they returned home. This occupational perspective could be included as part of the service users' initial and subsequent review meetings. During these initial assessments, the occupational therapist was able to establish with the service users what areas of occupation were important to them. Some people experienced great disruption to their occupational performance, while others had experienced a high degree of occupational deprivation in their daily life. This knowledge was significant in negotiating realistic goals with the service users and sharing this with the team. It also represented a positive way of defining occupational therapy in the acute setting.

The goals identified were often in conflict with the medical expectation of what the service user should achieve during admission or what would be possible to achieve on discharge; for example, if a person who usually lives on microwave meals and intends returning to this routine on discharge does not require a full assessment of cooking skills. Such an assessment would be of little value for the service user, and the occupational therapist could be doing something more meaningful with the service user. Although this assessment is often indicated, it is not seen as a priority by the service user as there is no risk involved in their current dietary intake.

Frustration in dealing with a service user in the hospital environment often comes from not having enough time, during a short stay, to address the issues that they identify. High levels of occupational alienation and deprivation are observed in service users. Working in a crisis intervention/home treatment team can allow time for more meaningful engagement with the service user in their home environment, doing activities that have real meaning for them in the context of their daily life. It could be argued that this intervention could be just as brief, but addressing these issues in response to the crisis could avert possible deterioration in engagement in occupation and ameliorate occupational alienation and deprivation.

Occupational therapists have the ability to work in these challenging areas of practice, but can they claim to be experts? In their opinion piece on consultant therapists, Craik and McKay (2003) suggest that an expert therapist should have practised in an area for more than 5 years. Such an expert would be able to function without direct reference to rules and procedures, would appear to view the whole picture intuitively and would have a vision of the possible and would be able to analyse complex situation and work towards resolutions. However, the development of expertise is not dependent on time alone. It requires active commitment to continuing professional development to further knowledge, extend skills and reflection on practice (College of Occupational Therapists, 2004).

Therapists often neglect to consider themselves as experts in their particular field of practice and that they have the ability to transfer their skills and knowledge into different working environments for the benefit of service users. Rather, they appear beset with issues of lack of confidence both as individual practitioners and as a profession. Occupational therapists can more easily identify the external sources of challenge – national policy, employers, management structures and institutional politics, but may not acknowledge their own internal challenges – lack of confidence in skills, fear of risk taking and limited vision of how occupational therapy can contribute in developing areas.

The delivery of health services is changing; non-traditional and extended-scope practice are becoming more commonplace, and health care is being defined not only by established health economies but also by the people who access the services. These changes compel individual therapists and the profession to consider new employment areas where therapists may work in roles that do not have occupational therapist in the title. Gage (1995) and Lloyd *et al.* (1999) discuss the adaptation required to keep occupational therapy relevant and core to changes in services. Pattison (2006) effectively proposes that occupational therapists need to act more as entrepreneurs in their approach and move the profession forward within the multitude of opportunities that these changes bring.

Now is the time for the profession to think creatively about ensuring that occupational therapy is available and delivered effectively to service users by thinking differently about how services can be delivered. With recent increases in the number of undergraduates being educated, there is an opportunity to move into role emerging posts. Negotiation with service managers to explore whether posts can be open to a range of professionals rather than being profession specific could allow occupational therapists entry to a service or allow for additional occupational therapy posts. This could also create more junior posts to build capacity and develop professional confidence and expertise in new areas of practice and provide opportunity for student placements, further developing the future workforce. Additionally, the profession must learn to take risks, whether they be big or small, and actively engage in new ways of working. This could be practising in non-traditional ways in statutory services and non-statutory services such as non-governmental and voluntary organisations.

Summary

There are many facets to this complex area of developing practice. Occupational therapists can contribute an occupational focus to working with service users at times of crisis. They understand that crisis is part of service users' illness experience, and engaging them in a client-centred manner at such time can assist them to retain and learn new skills, thus enabling them to continue with their recovery. Therapists have much to learn from service users especially in emerging practice areas such as crisis intervention. They are the key to ensuring that services really meet their needs; working in partnership with service users to lobby for changes is an effective way to improve practice.

To ensure that service users are able to benefit from occupational therapy, the profession has to be involved both at a practical and policy level. This contribution to crisis services should occur irrespective of whether occupational therapists work as specialists or more generically. However, it is important that the profession shapes strategic direction to maintain an occupational focus for service users in crisis.

There are undoubtedly challenges within this area of mental health practice because of the nature of working with service users at times of crisis. Occupational therapists need to be more proactive in engaging with these opportunities both at an individual and at a professional level. Occupational therapy has a responsibility to acknowledge its expertise and confidently transfer into extended scope practice.

Questioning your Practice

1. Can you identify ways that occupational therapy practice has developed as a result of the change in the delivery of services to individuals in crisis?
2. Would you consider yourself an 'expert' in your practice area?
3. How do we prove the effectiveness of occupational therapy to ensure service users and their carers benefit from occupation specific interventions during times of crisis?

References

Birchwood M, Smith J, Macmillan F, McGovern D (1998) Early Intervention in Psychotic Relapse. In: C Brooker, J Repper (eds) *Serious Mental Health Problems in the Community: Policy, Practice and Research.* London: Balliere Tindall.

Bowater J, Harrison M (2006) Implementing client-centred practice. *Occupational Therapy News, 14(4),* 35.

Brimblecombe N (2000) Suicidal ideation, home treatment and admission. *Mental Health Nursing, 20(1),* 22–26.

Campbell P (2000) Absence at the heart. *Openmind, (104),* 14–15.

Canadian Association of Occupational Therapists (1997) *Enabling Occupation: An Occupational Therapy Perspective.* Ottawa: CAOT Publications ACE.

Caplan G (1964) *Principles of Preventative Psychiatry.* London: Tavistock.

College of Occupational Therapists (2004) *Briefing 22 Competencies in Occupational Therapy.* London: COT.

Cook S (2003) Generic and specialist interventions for people with severe mental health problems: Can interventions be categorised? *British Journal of Occupational Therapy, 66(1),* 17–23.

Copeland ME (2001) Wellness recovery action plan: A system for monitoring, reducing and eliminating uncomfortable or dangerous physical symptoms and emotional feelings. In: C Brown (ed.) *Recovery and Wellness: Models of Hope and Empowerment for People with Mental Illness.* USA: The Haworth Press Inc., 127–150.

Craik C, McKay EA (2003) Consultant therapists: recognising and developing expertise. *British Journal of Occupational Therapy, 66(8),* 281–283.

Craik C, Austin C, Chacksfield JD, Richards G, Schell D (1998) College of Occupational Therapists: position paper on the way ahead for research, education and practice in mental health. *British Journal of Occupational Therapy, 61(9),* 390–395.

Creek J (2003) *OT defined as a complex intervention.* London: College of Occupational Therapists.

Dennis-Jones C (2005) Acute exodus in mental health. *Therapy Weekly,* 2 June 2005, 1.

Department of Health (2001) *The Mental Health Policy Implementation Guide.* London: DoH.

Dratcu L (2002) Acute hospital care: the beauty and the beast of psychiatry. *Psychiatric Bulletin, 26,* 81–82.

Duffy R, Nolan P (2005) A survey of the work of occupational therapists in inpatient mental health services. *Mental Health Practice, 8(6),* 36–41.

Ford R (1999) As you don't like it. *Health Services Journal,* 4 November 1999, 26–27.

Gage M (1995) Re-engineering of health care: Opportunity or threat for occupational therapists? *Canadian Journal of Occupational Therapy, 62(4),* 197–207.

Harrison M (2003) *Perceptions of Purpose and Outcome of Groups.* University of Birmingham: MA Community Mental Health.

Harrison M, Bahia I (2004) *Evaluation of Creative Activity Groups.* Sandwell Mental Health and Social Care Trust. Unpublished.

Harrison D (2003) The case for generic working in mental health occupational therapy. *British Journal of Occupational Therapy, 66(3),* 110–112.

Harries PA, Gilhooly K (2003) Generic and specialist occupational therapy casework in community mental health teams. *British Journal of Occupational Therapy, 66(3),* 101–109.

Harrison J, Alam N, Marshall J (2001) Home or away; which patients are suitable for a psychiatric home treatment service? *Psychiatric Bulletin, 25,* 310–313.

Hopkins C, Wasley S (2002) Intervening safely in a crisis. *Mental Health Nursing, 22(4),* 18–21.

Kielhofner G (2002) *A Model Of Human Occupation: Theory and Application.* (3rd edn) USA: Lippincott Williams and Wilkins.

Lane L (2000) Client Centred Practice: is it compatible with early discharge Hospital-at-Home Policies? *British Journal of Occupational Therapy, 63(7),* 310–315.

Lelliot P, Quirk A (2004) What is life really like on acute psychiatric wards? *Current Opinion in Psychiatry, (17),* 297–301.

Lloyd C, Kanowski H, Maas F (1999) Occupational therapy in mental health: challenges and opportunities. *Occupational Therapy International, 6(2),* 110–125.

Miller V, Robertson S (1991) A role for occupational therapy in crisis intervention and prevention. *Australian Occupational Therapy Journal, 38(3),* 143–146.

Onyett S (1998) *Case Management in Mental Health.* Cheltenham: Stanley Thornes (Publishers) Ltd.

Parker H (2001) The role of occupational therapists in community mental health teams: Generic or specialist? *British Journal of Occupational Therapy, 64(12),* 609–611.

Pattison M (2006) OT – outstanding talent: an entrepreneurial approach to practice. *Australian Occupational Therapy Journal, (58),* 166–172.

Polak PR, Kirby MW (1976) A model to replace psychiatric hospitals. *Journal of Nervous and Mental Disease, 162(1),* 13–22.

Reeves S, Summerfield Mann L (2004) Overcoming problems with generic working for occupational therapists based in community mental health settings. *British Journal of Occupational Therapy, 67(6),* 265–268.

Rosenfield MS (1984) Crisis intervention: the nuclear task approach. *American Journal of Occupational Therapy, 38(6),* 382–385.

Simpson A, Bowers L, Alexander J, Ridley C, Warren J (2005) Occupational therapy and multidisciplinary working on acute psychiatric wards: the Tompkins acute ward study. *British Journal of Occupational Therapy, 68(12),* 545–552.

Sumsion, T (2000) Client centred practice: The myths and realities. *Mental Health OT, 5(2),* 4–7.

Sumsion T (2005) Facilitating client-centred practice: Insights from clients. *Canadian Journal Of Occupational Therapy, 72(1),* 13–20.

Sumsion T (2006) *Client Centred Practice in Occupational Therapy: A Guide to Implementation.* 2nd edn. London: Churchill Livingstone.

The Mental Health Foundation (2003) *Project Summary: Improving Acute Psychiatric Hospital Services According to Inpatient Experiences.* London: The Mental Health Foundation.

The Sainsbury Centre for Mental Health (1998) *Acute Problems – A survey of the quality of care in acute psychiatric wards.* London: SCMH.

The Sainsbury Centre for Mental Health (2005) *Acute Care 2004: A National Survey of Adult Psychiatric Wards in England.* London: SCMH.

Yau MK (1995) Occupational therapy in community mental health: do we have a unique role in the interdisciplinary environment? *Australian Occupational Therapy Journal, 42(3),* 129–132.

6 'Doing' in secure settings

Elaine Hunter and Elizabeth Anne McKay

Personal narrative

My work as an occupational therapist began when I was a student in York. I qualified in 1985 and then began practising in Edinburgh. Throughout my career I have always worked in mental health settings in Scotland, first in a rehabilitation day unit for people with enduring and severe mental illness and in acute care both for people under and over 65 years. Latterly, I have practised in a range of secure units initially on an intensive psychiatric care unit and then in a medium secure forensic unit, but more about that later. I am a clinician and a manager and I believe strongly in the principles of developing an evidence-based, client centred-service enabling the potential and social inclusion of individuals.

Until recently I was the professional lead for occupational therapy in a primary care trust in Scotland, with approximately 140 occupational therapists employed in all aspects of service delivery in learning disabilities, rehabilitation and mental health services incorporating acute admissions, vocational rehabilitation and specialist services including child and adolescent mental health, substance misuse and homeless practice.

As both a practitioner and manager, I have always valued supervision in my professional life. This interest led me to explore supervision in occupational therapy in mental health for my BSc in Health Studies (Hunter, 1991) and then the implementation of a supervision package for all staff (Hunter & Blair, 1999). Currently I am completing a Master's in Occupational Therapy and this has allowed me to examine the implementation of evidence-based practice in the allied health professions and the role of the manager. This work is in its early stages and will be reported in due course.

As a student I was fortunate to be taught by Linda Finlay, and I developed an interest in group and personal awareness and completed two group analytic courses over 3 consecutive years. Although these courses did not lead to formal qualifications, they provided a valuable learning experience of the importance of reflecting and listening, not just to what people say but how they say it. I have also had 10 years' experience of being a facilitator in group analysis within a psychotherapy outpatient service using the principles of Foulkes (1964).

Over the last few years I have become a mother of two young sons who keep me busy in lots of ways and have given me the greatest learning curve of my life, as there are no textbooks that tell you how you will respond to being a working mother or the overwhelming feeling of pleasure when your children make small steps in their development.

I now work in a medium secure forensic psychiatry setting, the interface between mental health services and the criminal justice system. Clients may have acute or chronic mental health difficulties, personality disorder, problems with substance misuse or a combination of these. They may have committed or been charged with a criminal offence or their mental illness is unmanageable in normal prison contexts. In this chapter, when case examples are given, there will be mention of an index offence. The details of these have not been included to ensure the confidentiality of the clients, but readers need to be aware that a crucial factor of forensic service is that, when an offence has been committed, 'for the most part these assaults are against victims they already know: wives, children, relatives, friends or neighbours' (Higgens, 1995, p. 57). So when considering clients' and professionals' narratives, their sense of loss can be overwhelming.

As forensic mental health settings increase, this area of practice tests occupational therapists. The clients may have limited 'occupational abilities, their choices and opportunities have often been eroded due to the effects of long-term institutionalisation' (Cronin-Davies *et al.*, 2004, p. 170). Furthermore, some individuals are affected by earlier experiences including the contexts in which they grew up and lived. Mountain (1998) reminds us that that the range of problems, people with a forensic history exhibit, is wide and complex.

Given this background, this chapter will explore the use of narrative as a means for creating meaningful occupational engagement in the forensic setting. Some of the narratives come from the team members I now supervise.

Introduction to forensic psychiatry in Scotland

Flood (1997) identified five settings for forensic services in the UK: maximum secure hospitals, medium secure hospitals, low secure hospitals, private secure hospitals and prisons. In Scotland, The State Hospital at Carstairs provides maximum secure services for Scottish and Northern Irish patients. The early special hospitals throughout the UK were isolated both geographically, to some extent, socially and professionally and their values and practices went largely unchallenged (Nolan, 2005).

The Butler Report (Home Office and Department of Health and Social Security, 1975) was influential in the establishment of regional secure units within the mental health sector, although not in Scotland. The Reed Report (Department of Health and Home Office, 1992) reviewed the current services available for mentally disordered offenders and stressed that local services were crucial. However, until 2001, in Scotland, forensic psychiatry was mainly practised in local intensive care units of psychiatric hospitals, in some out-patient facilities and by The State Hospital at Carstairs – no unit met the recognised medium secure standards as outlined by the Scottish Executive (2006).

A number of crucial reports influenced services in Scotland. The Scottish Office document 'Health, social work and related services for mentally disordered offenders in Scotland' (1999) provided guiding principles similar to the earlier Reed report proposing that 'Health boards should investigate the need for a structured development of local facilities and services to provide for mentally disordered offenders from courts, prisons and returning from The State Hospital' (p. 29). Despite this directive, there was no funding recommendations or allocations available.

However, one primary care trust in Scotland had an aspiration to re-provide hospital services, and in conjunction with a number of lead clinicians, proposed a new forensic medium secure unit gaining Scottish Office approval in May 1999. This unit serves a population of 1.5 million people, covering the geographical area of southeast Scotland. The unit is located within the grounds of the mental health hospital for the city of Edinburgh, the Royal Edinburgh Hospital; it has 50 forensic beds, 25 acute medium secure and 25 long-term medium secure beds. Clients are admitted from the courts, prisons and The State Hospital.

The new forensic unit is small, and the staff adopts approaches to their work that are similar to those in use by health care personnel elsewhere. However, the historical tension in forensic services between care and containment had also to be considered (Porter, 2002). Special reference was given to the different power dynamics in forensic mental health outlined by Nolan (2005, p.14), who states there is a 'dominance of the biomedical model' sustained 'through its close alliance with the law, while psychology has sought to assert itself through the alliance with research and education'. Nolan (2005) suggests that team meetings and discussions cannot mask the lack of genuine parity among the staff groups. This is supported by Coffey and Jenkins (2002), who note that consultants have a statutory role of responsible medical officer and social workers have a statutory responsibility as social supervisors, unlike nurses and occupational therapists who may be excluded from key decision-making processes. In designing the building and the service, it was also necessary to acknowledge these factors and work with the reality of clinical practice and in partnership with everyone involved, including the team and clients who access the service.

As Head Occupational Therapist in the Intensive Psychiatric Care Unit (IPCU) the brief in 1999 was to develop and design an occupational therapy service for the first medium secure unit in Scotland, The Orchard Clinic. The design process was exciting but detailed with hours spent deliberating over items like the depth of the doors to the heights of the perimeter fence.

In the design process, consideration was given to the clients' current and future needs and to the scope of occupational therapy within this environment. The design of the therapy facility concentrated on the environment, making good use of natural light, developing, as much as possible, a non-institutional setting, creating rooms that were spacious and would allow creativity and choice but at all times be secure. It was also important that the design, both of the building and philosophy of practice, could be integrated with the occupational therapists in the wider mental health service to ensure ease of access to services for the clients. After extensive consultation and hard work by the multi-disciplinary team, this unit admitted its first patients in January 2001. Two further medium secure units will open in Scotland, in 2007 for the West of Scotland and Glasgow and in 2011 for the North of Scotland.

Occupational therapy in forensic settings

Couldrick (2003, p. 13) suggests that forensic occupational therapy 'can be seen not only as the treatment of people with mental health problems who offend but also as a means of addressing offending behaviour'. It is about acknowledging the important link between occupational behaviour and well-being.

Forensic services care for some of the most marginalised, vulnerable and difficult-to-treat individuals in society. Those admitted to forensic facilities may spend an average of 18 months as in-patients and, in some cases, in excess of 3 years. Such psychiatric clients take longer to rehabilitate for reasons of chronicity and legal status. Today, the concept of forensic care can still evoke negative feelings in people who are normally rational and fair minded (Nolan, 2005). Thomspen et al. (1999) highlighted that staff, too, can be repulsed by forensic patients and their behaviour. Lloyd (1995) highlights 'the client group itself is not an easy group to work with' (p. 210).

Case Study 6.1 Negative feelings

I work with Stephen who has never acknowledged his index offence or indeed his mental health illness. My role was initially to consider how he spent his day and what occupations would be meaningful for him in this setting. However, it became clear in working with him that he evoked negative feelings in some of the staff. He interacted with the majority of staff in a derogatory manner using sarcastic and discriminatory comments, creating many negative transference situations. It was apparent that he responded well to staff in a hierarchy position within the clinic. When I worked with Stephen, I was aware of his negative responses towards staff that could then result in undermining comments from some staff. It was therefore crucial to be aware of his limited insight into his mental illness and into his own negative communication.

This example highlights that it is essential for good staff support, time to reflect and a supervision structure to be available. Regardless of the apparent challenges of individual histories, and the obtrusive security measures in forensic settings, Crawford and Mee (1994) emphasised that the occupational therapy process is the same as in psychiatric settings elsewhere. Chacksfield (1997) agreed, but he highlighted additional aspects to be considered, including safer environment and security, level of knowledge of mental health legislation and patients' knowledge of their rights. Flood (1997) stressed that other factors can also impact on occupational therapy. For example, activities can be limited because of the secure environment; access to resources or equipment maybe restricted and attendance at activities may be reliant on sufficient staff to provide adequate cover. Finally, patients' motivation may be reduced because of their perception of being confined against their will.

That said, Cronin-Davies *et al.* (2004, p. 170) stated that it is important to 'acknowledge that the nature of secure environments can limit patients' access to a diverse range of occupations, which might be available to them in other settings'. The challenges that face occupational therapists working in forensic areas are two-fold: the first is the ever-present risk posed by patients and second is the need to be resourceful and creative in facilitating occupational engagement relevant to these risks. Despite this challenge, the work is satisfying when the clients do leave the clinic and, with the right support, move to their own accommodation. Two colleagues from The Orchard Clinic published a short report 'From Seedling to Service' and wrote ' in our opinion, working with the clients is the highlight of the day, being able to offer them an activity that they are interested in, and will assist them with their recovery is extremely rewarding' (Schofield and Spencely, 2006, p. 23).

Most occupational therapy intervention in a forensic setting is focused on enabling individuals to attain skills in daily living tasks, vocational and social skills, enabling them to be reintegrated, into the community. To achieve these goals, a key skill of the occupational therapist is the ability to engage and motivate patients by using a diversity of occupations tailored to meet their specific needs, skills and aspirations. While it is the ultimate aim of occupational therapy to enable individuals to experience occupational enrichment and achieve occupational functioning, it can be hugely challenging within secure environments, and so the occupational therapist's skill is in devising creative and versatile treatment programmes with and for their clients.

Case Study 6.2   Being creative

During a peer review, a therapist presented a client (Jim), who, after completing an interest checklist, stated that he had a strong interest in learning Spanish. However, the occupational therapist's role was to prepare him for discharge from the clinic and, in particular, budgeting skills. Jim, however, showed little interest in looking at budgeting. He had been in an institutional setting for many years and learning Spanish did not appear to relate to the clinic's role of assisting him in the basic skills of living. However, with some thought and creativity, the therapist introduced the use of the computer to assist Jim to learn his Spanish and was then able to use this skill to look at budgeting on the computer. By listening to Jim's interests to learn Spanish, the therapist gained his trust to focus on his improving his much-needed budgeting skills on a limited budget.

Maximising the evidence base

The early literature on forensic occupational therapy describes interventions with few examples of evaluating specific treatment (Lloyd, 1983, 1995; Chacksfield,

1997; Flood, 1997; Forward *et al.*, 1999). A review by Mountain (1998) emphasised the requirement for consolidation and development of the existing evidence base in forensic occupational therapy. This noted an overall paucity of material with research having been undertaken as individual projects in specific areas of interest rather than a result of a strategic decision (Mountain, 1998).

The College of Occupational Therapists has gone some way to address this by publishing the *Research and Development Strategic Vision and Action Plan for Forensic Occupational Therapists* (COT, 2002). This report set six objectives over a 10-year period. The forensic strategic vision suggests all practitioners be research aware and suggests establishing posts with a dedicated research/continuing professional development component. Duncan *et al.* (2003) also highlighted research as a priority for forensic psychiatry. A further paper by the College of Occupational Therapists (2003) for forensic occupational therapy in residential setting supports the need for an evidence base to underpin the framework for occupational therapy practice from which models of practice are devised. The challenge remains for relevant and strategic research in forensic psychiatry to be conducted.

When reviewing occupational therapy in forensic settings, there is some published research including the work by Garner *et al.* (1996), Baker and McKay (2001) and Gooch and Living (2004). However, evidence has been used in the clinical service during monthly peer reviews – these reviews involve occupational therapy staff and students to assist reflection on the narratives and needs of the clients. Three research reports have been vital in this process: Clarke (2002), Farnworth *et al.* (2004) and Mason (2006).

The work by Clarke (2002) was an unpublished study to determine the extent to which forensic mental health service users were involved in decisions regarding their care, and it examined their desired involvement in the decision-making process. She looked at the impact on culture within the forensic service and on residents' involvement in decision making. The findings demonstrated that, where residents' current and desired involvement was strongly influenced by the culture and where staff had negative perceptions of residents, the level of resident involvement was diminished (p. 72).

Case Study 6.3 Culture and user involvement

During the peer review, staff considered the clinic culture and the need for management to promote a culture of user involvement in care planning and the provision of information. This led to two therapists and a social work colleague meeting with the patients' council and reviewing the literature on user involvement. From this work, they established a user advocacy group available to all the clients in the clinic, and it will have formal links to the clinic management team. This initiative is still in its infancy but gives a focus for a culture of trying to listen to clients on the environment in which they live.

Farnworth *et al.* (2004) studied how the in-patients of a secure forensic psychiatric facility in Australia used their time and viewed their opportunities for occupational engagement in this environment. They found that time use was dominated by personal care and leisure occupations and the participants were dissatisfied with their time use, describing themselves as 'bored' or 'killing time'. The article drew on the idea that learning about people's prior occupations and life experiences contributed to understanding their present occupational choices and interests and the meanings that they ascribed to occupations. The conclusion was that a more systematic use of tools, such as OPHI-II in forensic settings might help staff to identify the opportunities for occupational engagement that use the personal resources of individuals within specific groups offered and within the overall residential environment.

Case Study 6.4 Occupational histories

This peer review challenged me to reflect on how and if I offer choice in therapy and it reaffirmed the need to give the opportunity to hear and understand an individual's occupational history. Within the clinic, the OPHI-II is used and this supported the need for its continued use. The article confirmed the importance of the client's previous experiences and positive relationships to their motivation to engage and sustain involvement.

The unpublished thesis by Mason (2006) was conducted in a high-security unit and examined the factors that influence engagement in therapeutic group work. She identified two themes about participant's engagement in therapeutic group work. The most significant and far-reaching influence was the culture of the environment and the other was the concept of choice, which stems from and is greatly influenced by the first.

Case Study 6.5 Engagement in groups

This thesis was presented in a peer review to the team and gave the opportunity to reflect on the current groups provided and to consider if enough choice was offered. It raised further questions: Is the environment stimulating? Are clients asked their opinion on treatment options? Is enough emphasis placed on the aims of the groups in the clinic and should every group provided over the year be peer-reviewed?

These case studies do not critically appraise the evidence; they aim to explore how professional narratives can challenge thinking within a peer-review culture. Evidence in occupational therapy and in the developing academic field of occupational science has also been considered.

The influence of occupational science

There have been times when the staff group has looked to occupational therapy when they perceive a patient to be 'bored'. Clinical teams have referred patients because they are bored, and this leads to the question 'Why do people engage in occupation and what are the influencing factors?'

Occupational science has examined the relationship between health and occupation. Wilcock (1991) defines occupational science as the 'systematic study of all aspects of the relationship between humans and occupation, occupation encompassing peoples goal directed use of time, energy, interest and attention in work, leisure, family, cultural, self care and rest activities' (p. 297).

Farnworth (1998) considered boredom in her research with young offenders on probation. Significantly more boredom was experienced when they were engaged in passive leisure and personal care occupations and was less likely to occur when they engaged in education or active leisure occupations. The implementation of flow theory is important for the therapist to facilitate the challenge of an occupation to be equal or more to the skills the individual client brings to the situation.

The theory of flow is important when considering occupational engagement. Rebeiro and Polgar (1999) suggest that understanding it assists appreciation of human occupation. Csikszentimihalyi (1975) (cited in Emerson, 1998, p. 38) defined flow as 'a subjective psychological state, which occurs when one is totally in an activity'. Flow is the 'total involvement in what one is doing with a high degree of emotional satisfaction which continually attracts people to challenging occupations' (Yerxa, 1993, p. 7). Rebeiro and Polgar (1999) suggest that matching challenge and skills is important; however, if the challenge is greater than the individual's skills, then anxiety will result, and if the individual skills are greater than those required of the activity, boredom will result.

Cronin-Davis *et al.* (2004) suggest that occupational science can be used to guide occupational therapy assessment and treatment and inform the developing area of forensic practice. It provides a theoretical framework that enables therapists to explore and understand the complexities of engaging patients in meaningful occupation. This offers alternative perspectives when working with clients who appear unmotivated or when engagement breaks down.

Viewing clients as occupational beings can be especially effective in such environments. This perspective requires that the occupational therapy assessment establish, the causes of occupational dysfunction, in particular to identify the occupational risk factors impacting on the individual. These risk factors include performance deficits, occupational disruption, occupational imbalance, occupational deprivation, occupational alienation or a combination of these.

This is critical in an in-patient forensic setting, where there are many restrictions on clients – for the therapeutic safety of clients and staff, doors being locked, meals being at a set time and restricted access to the community.

Furthermore, to understand a client and his or her motivation occupational science advocates listening to peoples' stories. Narrative, it is proposed, is the primary form by which human experience is made meaningful (Polkinghorne, 1988). As personal meaning is offered through the individual's narrative, Mattingly (1998) considers the narrative form particularly appropriate for addressing illness and healing experiences. For clients in forensic settings, understanding their life stories and their journeys through an institutional system is vital; their illness may be overshadowed by their index crime. In narrative terms, the 'illness or disability' is considered an episode within the larger context of the individual's life history.

Mattingly (1998) regards narratives as being 'event and experience-centred, which create experiences for the listener or audience' (p. 8). Williams (1984) posits that during certain times of crisis, the life story is disrupted or lost. The routine narrative can become confused, resulting in some reworking of the narrative to account for the disruption. This reconstruction is necessary 'in order to understand the illness in terms of past social experience and to reaffirm that life has a course and the self a purpose' (p. 179). Such stories hold our experiences together, allowing links to the past, present and, crucially, to the future. This is vital for occupational therapy and client-centred practice.

Case Study 6.6 Life story

When I first heard Grace's life story, I saw a woman who had many roles in her life: daughter, wife, mother, colleague, friend and, now, patient. When living at home, she had a relapse of her mental illness; she became very unwell and was untreated. This led her to the index offence and its desperate consequences resulting in her becoming a forensic in-patient.

Working with Grace, thinking with her and listening to her life history enabled me to see the woman she was and to work with her to help her find a road to recovery that gave her the opportunity to re-establish some of her life roles and to live with the consequence of her index offence.

Strategies and interventions: individual or group work?

When applying the evidence base and the principles of occupation in forensic psychiatry, the constant question is what is best – individual work or treatment groups? Striving for a mixture of the two approaches seems the best option.

With individual work, it is crucial to remember that the importance of the interpersonal relationship with clients cannot be underestimated and it is the quality of relationships formed with staff that is the strongest determinant of successful outcome (Nolan *et al.*, 1999). To assist the development of individual work, practice is guided by incorporating the Model of Human Occupation (Kielhofner, 1980), a frequently used model in a forensic setting (Duncan *et al.*, 2003). The assessments available from this model assist the consideration of the client's client's life history, motivation and how the client spends their day and utilise their time.

Within the first week of admission, wherever possible, a patient will have contact with an occupational therapist, when a risk assessment is completed along with an interest checklist and a programme of occupation. The Model of Human Occupation Screening Tool (MOHOST; Parkinson *et al.*, 2006) is used as a baseline assessment with other standardised assessments as required.

The occupational therapist working with the client would determine the appropriate use of specific assessments or reassessments based on the clinical judgement of the therapist, problems identified through observation or other assessments, observed changes in level of functioning, client's needs and the outcome of specific intervention. It is clear that certain attributes are necessary including good clinical skills, a natural curiosity, tolerance of difficult behaviour, balanced attitude towards offending behaviour, ability to communicate, ability to seek support and a sense of humour (Chiswick, 1995; Dale, 2001).

The provision of group work is a challenge for all staff. Couldrick (2003) writes:

> *I suspect most seasoned forensic occupational therapists have experienced times when the whole activity programme has collapsed. Not only must occupational therapists be able to motivate the client, he or she must also be able to re-motivate themselves. (p. 18)*

This outlines the constant struggle to maintain groups, and this is managed in a number of ways. The first way is to have a leader but with a multi-disciplinary focus. The second is that a group treatment is integral to the culture of the clinic and that all group interventions are respected by all, form the quiz group right through to the Cognitive Behavior Therapy (CBT) anger management group.

There is a consistent approach in the clinic amongst staff to ensure that there is a clear and common language about group work familiar to all team members. The model used is based on Finlay's (1994, 1997) classification of groups in occupational therapy and adapted for a multi-disciplinary and user focus. Finlay distinguishes between activity task and social-based groups, and support-based groups that include communication and psychotherapy or a mixture of the two. The classification describes groups having an aim, therapeutic focus and orientation ranging from end product to group processes. These groups are innovative and creative, ranging from treatment of addictions and carers support group to art therapy, music therapy, life skills, gardening group and a yearly photography exhibition. Clients' perspectives on groups are sought through an audit of all the groups, on a cyclical basis.

Case Study 6.7   A lunch group in a medium secure setting

This lunch group is run for the acute ward with the purpose of providing a group through the normal activity of making lunch. The group aims and motivates clients through a sense of achievement. Two experienced therapists facilitate it, and frequently there are occupational therapy students on placement as this group is a good learning environment; here a student was present.

The kitchen is large, non-institutional, painted in a bright turquoise colour with access to tea or coffee, the choice of having the radio on or off and to join in the activity or sit and watch. This particular group had five clients: four men and one woman, and all had been in the group for at least 1 month to over 2 years. There were a variety of needs to cater for because of the range of skills and time in the clinic.

Two of the group had come from the courts, one from prison and two from The State Hospital. The future for all participants was unclear and uncertain with the potential of one returning to prison, one awaiting an appearance at court and three to be discharged from the clinic but with no potential discharge date in sight. Serious offences had brought them into contact with the service and all had their own stories of disruptive childhoods and long-term mental health problems, but with some level of support from families. As a result of the uncertainty of each group member, although they were all in the same room with the same task, to cook and eat their lunch, they were five individuals, and it is for the occupational therapist to ensure the group is safe both environmentally and psychologically.

(Continued)

Case Study 6.7 Continued

They cook, chat, eat, plan for the next week and then they return to their wards. However, during that hour and a half, the therapist listens to the clients' stories. Through their stories, it becomes apparent how important this group is to them. One of the clients frequently states that it breaks up his day and he becomes 'bored' when there are no 'classes' on. For another patient, the role of cooking is a skill he values as this was his previous role, and he takes great pride in speaking about the restaurants that he has worked in. The group offers him the opportunity to reflect on his past achievements and previous identity. The youngest and newest member of the group appears anxious, and talks constantly, but he speaks with great delight of recipes he knows and wishes to share with his peer group. Although he appears anxious in the group, he continues to attend, and it is hoped that over time this group may become a place for him to relax. There is a quiet member in the group who always watches what is being cooked, but this is the only group he will attend on a regular basis and he always assists in deciding what should be cooked. There is one member for whom being in the kitchen is a reminder of a negative role outside the clinic and he does not take an active part, will not eat the cooked food and, it is anticipated, will not continue to attend. But attending is important until he will engage in an occupation that he would value more.

When working in this setting, awareness of current and historical risk assessment is important, but this should not detract from the therapist becoming involved in listening to what occupations mean to the patients and the role they take. During and after each session the therapist must think about the role as a mentor to the other therapist and as educator to the student.

When sharing these ideas, the theory of guided reflection proposed by Johns (2000) is used; this is composed of a series of questions, arranged in a logical order, that help the reflective practitioner tune into an experience. The model commences by 'Looking in', which encourages the practitioner to pause amidst the hectic pace of life and find a quiet space to focus on thoughts and feelings. The main part is 'Looking out', which offers a series of thoughts and feelings and reflective cues to focus the practitioner's attention on significant issues within the experience. After each session, staff and students think about what happened in the group and reflect on their role and the stories they have heard during the group.

To conclude, working in forensic settings requires occupational therapists to gain understanding of an individual's unique occupational history to enable sensitive and creative occupational therapy to be delivered as part of the rehabilitation process. The importance of continual review through supervision and reflection of professional practice and the developing evidence base is essential to meet the challenge of these contexts.

Questioning your practice

1. What evidence is shaping your own practice?
2. In your setting what mechanisms exist to review practice and evidence and to make changes?
3. In what ways do you reflect on your work experiences?

References

Baker S, McKay E (2001) Occupational therapists perspectives on the needs of woman in medium secure units. *British Journal of Occupational Therapy, 67(10)*, 441–448.

Chiswick D (1995) Introduction. In: D Chiswick , R Cope (eds) *Practical Forensic Psychiatry*. Trowbridge: Redwood Press, 1–13.

Chacksfield JD (1997) Forensic occupational therapy: is it a developing specialism? *British Journal of Therapy and Rehabilitation, 4(7)*, 371–374.

Clarke C (2002) Current and desired involvement of forensic mental health service users in decisions regarding their care. Advanced Programme in Occupational Therapy, St Loye's School of Health Sciences: Unpublished MSc Thesis.

Coffey M, Jenkins E (2002) Power and control: forensic community mental health nurses perceptions of team working, legal sanctions and compliance. *Journal of Psychiatric and Mental Health Nursing, 9(5)*, 553–562.

College of Occupational Therapists (2002) *Research and Department Strategic Vision and Action Plan.*

College of Occupational Therapists (2003) *Standards of Practice for Occupational Therapy in Forensic Residential Settings.* January. London: COT.

College of Occupational Therapists (2007) *Recovering Ordinary Lives. The Strategy for Occupational Therapy in Mental Health Services 2007–2017 Literature Review.* London: COT.

Couldrick L (2003) So what is forensic occupational therapy? In: L Couldrick, D Alfred (eds) *Forensic Occupational Therapy*. London: Whurr Publishers, Chapter 2, 11–21.

Crawford M, Mee J (1994) The role of occupational therapy in the rehabilitation of the mentally disordered offender. *British Journal of Occupational Therapy, 57(1)*, 293–294.

Cronin-Davis J, Lang A, Molineux M (2004) Occupational Science: The Forensic Challenge. In: M Molineux (ed.) *Occupation for Occupational Therapists*. Oxford: Blackwell Publishing Ltd, 169–179.

Dale C (2001) Interpersonal relationships: Staff development, awareness and monitoring issues. In: C Dale, T Thompson, P Woods (eds) *Forensic Mental Health Issues in Practice* . Edinburgh: Bailiere Tindall.

Department of Health and Home Office (1992) *Review of Health and Social Services for Mentally Disordered Offenders and Others Requiring Similar Services* final summary report chaired by Dr John Reid, London: HMSO.

Duncan EAS, Munro K, Nicol MM (2003) Research priorities in forensic occupational therapy. *British journal of Occupational Therapy, 66(2)*, 55–63.

Emerson H (1998) Flow and occupation: A review of the literature. *Canadian Journal of Occupational Therapy 65(1)*, 37–44.

Farnworth L (1998) Doing, being and boredom. *Journal of Occupational Science, 5(3)*, 140–146.

Farnworth L, Nikitin L, Fossey E (2004) Being in a secure forensic psychiatric Unit: Every Day is the same. Killing time or making the most of it. *British Journal of Occupational Therapy, 67(10)*, 430–438.

Finlay L (1994) *Groupwork in Occupational Therapy*. London: Chapman & Hall.

Finlay L (1997) Groupwork. In: J Creek (ed.) *Occupational Therapy and Mental Health*. Edinburgh: Churchill Livingstone.

Flood B (1997) An introduction to occupational therapy in forensic psychiatry. *British Journal of Therapy and Rehabilitation*, 4(7), 375–380.

Forward MJ, Lloyd C, Trevan-Hawke J (1999) Occupational therapy in the forensic psychiatric setting. *British Journal of Therapy and Rehabilitation, 6(9)*, 442–446.

Foulkes SH (1964) *Therapeutic Group Analysis*. Woking: Unwin Brothers Limited.

Garner R, Butler G, Hutchings D (1996) Study of the relationship between the patterns of planned activity and incidents of deliberate self-harm within a regional secure unit. *British Journal of Occupational Therapy, 59(4)*, 156–160.

Gooch P, Living R (2004) The therapeutic use of videogames within secure forensic settings: A review of the literature and application to practice. *British Journal of Occupational Therapy, 67(8),* 332–341.

Higgins J (1995) Crime and mental disorder II. Forensic aspects of psychiatric disorder. In: D Chiswick, R Cope eds . *Practical Forensic Psychiatry.* Trowbridge: Redwood Press.

Home Office and Department of Health and Social Security (1975) *Report of the Committee on Mentally Abnormal Offenders (Butler Report).* London: HMSO.

Hunter EP (1991) Support and supervision for occupational therapy staff working in mental health. Queen Margaret College, Edinburgh: Unpublished BSc Dissertation.

Hunter EP, Blair SEE (1999) Staff supervision for occupational therapists. *British Journal of Occupational Therapy, 62(8),* 344–350.

Johns C (2000) *Becoming a Reflective Practitioner: A reflective and holistic Approach to Clinical Nursing, Practice Development and Clinical Supervision.* Edinburgh: Blackwell Science.

Kielhofner G (1980) A model of human occupation, Part 2. Ontogenesis from the perspective of temporal adaptation. *American Journal of Occupational Therapy, 34,* 657–663.

Lloyd C (1983) Forensic psychiatry and occupational therapy. *British Journal of Occupational Therapy, 47,* 348–350.

Lloyd C (1995) Trends in forensic psychiatry. *British Journal of Occupational Therapy, 58(5),* 209–213.

Mason K (2006) Factors that influence engagement in therapeutic group-work within a high security hospital environment: male patient perspectives. Middlesex University: Unpublished MSc thesis.

Mattingly C (1998) *Healing Dramas and Clinical Plots: The Narrative structure of Experience.* Cambridge: Cambridge University Press.

Parkinson S, Forsyth K, Keilhofner G (2006) *The Model of Human Occupation Screening Tool* (MOHOST) Version 2.0. http://www.moho.uic.edu/assess/mohost.html. Accessed 28 March 2006.

Mountain G (1998) *Occupational therapy in forensic settings. A preliminary review of the knowledge and research base,* London: College of Occupational Therapy.

Nolan P (1999) The historical context. In: S Wix, M Humphreys *(eds) Multidisciplinary Working in Forensic Mental Health Care.* Edinburgh: Elsevier Churchill Livingstone.

Nolan P (2005) Historical context In: SH Wix, M Humprheys, 2005. Multi-disciplinary working in foresic Mental Health Care Elsvier Churchil Livingstone, Chapter 1.

Polkinghorne DE (1988) *Narrative Knowing and the Human Sciences.* Albany, NY: State University of New York Press.

Porter R (2002) *Madness, A Brief History.* Oxford: Oxford University Press.

Rebeiro, K., & Miller Polgar, J. (1999). Enabling occupational performance: Optimal experiences in therapy. *Canadian Journal of Occupational Therapy, 66(1),* 14–22.

Schofield P, Spenceley H (2006) From seedling to service. *Occupational Therapy News, 14(4),* 23.

Scottish Office (1999) *Health, Social Work and Related Services for Mentally Disordered Offenders in Scotland.* NHS MEL 5.

Scottish Executive (2006) *Forensic Mental Health Services* NHS HDL (2006) 48. Forensic Mental Health Managed Care Network, www.forensicnetwork.scot.nhs.uk

Thomspen S, Soares J, Nolan P, Dallender J, Arnetz B (1999) Feelings of professional fulfilment and exhaustion in mental health personnel: the Importance of organisational and individual factors. *Psychotherapy and Psychosomatics, 68,* 157–164.

Wilcock AA (1998) *An Occupational Perspective of Health.* Thorofare, NJ: Slack Incorporated.

Wilcock AA (1991) Occupational science. *British Journal of Occupational Therapy, 54(8),* 297–300.

Williams G (1984) The genesis of chronic illness: narrative reconstruction. *Sociology of Health and Illness, 6(2),* 175–200.

Yerxa E (1993) Occupational Science: a new source of power for participants in occupational therapy. *Occupational Science Australia, 1(1),* 3–10.

7 Occupational, social and intrapersonal alienation explored in the community

Wendy Bryant

Personal narrative

My dream was to be an artist; however, this was seen by my family as indulgent and economically risky. So I became an occupational therapist, bringing with me a curiosity about multiple meanings of experiences. I was especially curious about mental illness, having explored the work of Jung whilst studying at school (Jung *et al.*, 1995). The bridge he suggested between symbols and intrapersonal psychology was something I wanted to continue to explore .

Immersed in Jung, in 1980 I had my first experience of psychiatry when I visited the hospital where a friend had been admitted. I went to see the occupational therapy department, which was also home to a rabbit, and I was struck by the image of the caged animal in an asylum. I met an occupational therapy student there, and she warned me 'don't think this is occupational therapy, it's not' and I was puzzled to know the difference. It looked as if the people in the department were better off than the ones outside, roaming the grounds or behind the grey walls and windows of the wards. These thoughts stayed with me as I progressed through the course, qualifying in 1984. Over the next 18 years I worked mainly as a senior occupational therapist in hospitals and in the community, in mental health and physical disability settings. I did some research (Bryant, 1991, 1995; Bryant *et al.* 2004, 2005), had two children and continued to work part time as they grew up.

My overriding passion has been to explore how people who are routinely silenced and ignored in everyday care settings can be given a voice. This emphasis on the everyday is critical. My practice and research must impact the everyday to make a difference. This means exploring multiple interpretations of experience, just as I have done as an artist. There are many ways to paint a portrait and there are many ways for people to express their hopes. Enabling people to do this involves working in a risky, creative way. This is what has kept me an occupational therapist. I have found that one of the most satisfying ways of exploring multiple interpretations is to do research.

My first experience of working in the community mental health setting was when the NHS and Community Care Act (1990) was beginning to impact on services. I spent half my time working with individuals requiring short-term interventions and the other half of my time developing day services in the local area for people with longer-term problems. The expectation was that day services would take place in the local community. There were two beliefs in relation to this. The first belief was that people would use them as a stepping stone to being involved in the community, eventually feeling confident and well enough to belong to other groups that were open to everyone. The second belief was that professional involvement was required only initially to get the day services going and foster an emphasis on social contact and meaningful occupation. It was important not to create dependency, and so I was expected to share responsibility with service users for leading the services.

These beliefs reflected the government policies of the 1980s, which built on a political and clinical desire to increase community services, justified both in terms of economics and deinstitutionalisation. My post involved balancing resources between people newly referred and those who used services over the long term. At the time, the main way of engaging with long-term service users in the community was through out-patient appointments with psychiatrists, depot injections or day services. The views that day services were a stepping stone to the community, or would become service user led, were challenged by this group of people. Many were already known in the community and, at best, had established social networks. They knew far more about the local community than I did, and what they valued was the opportunity to meet with each other. Research at the time reflected this (Brewer *et al.*, 1994; Bryant, 1995).

These issues arose again in my master's research (Bryant *et al.*, 2004, 2005) and the concept of occupational alienation emerged as a useful foundation for further exploration. This chapter explores occupational alienation (Wilcock, 1998) pointing to the absence of creativity and meaning in occupation as a factor in mental ill health. I believe that the current emphasis on the outcomes of interventions, rather than the processes, generates increased occupational alienation for service users.

Occupational alienation defined

Occupational alienation has been defined as a 'sense of isolation, powerlessness, frustration, loss of control, and estrangement from society or self as a result of engagement in occupation that does not satisfy inner needs' (Wilcock, 2006, p. 343). The concept was proposed by Wilcock (1998) in relation to the theory that health was dependent on a person engaging in meaningful occupations. She considered what might interfere with this process, identifying the occupational risk factors of occupational deprivation, alienation and imbalance.

Occupational therapists in the USA also sought to develop an occupational perspective explaining ill health in terms of occupation (Zemke & Clark, 1996; Yerxa, 2000). This occupational perspective demanded a broader definition of occupation, to incorporate everything a person does in his or her life (Wilcock, 1998). From this standpoint, it was possible to look at how the things people do shape their identity and roles in social contexts. It also enabled environmental factors to be acknowledged as determinants of occupational performance.

Wilcock's (1998) conception of occupational alienation emphasised that demands of everyday life required people to do things that lacked personal meaning, such as boring and repetitive tasks that isolate people from each other (Wilcock, 2006). Embedded in this are three elements:

■ absence of personal meaning or meaninglessness, an internal state;
■ absence of opportunities to be creative and control meaningful occupations and tasks;
■ social isolation or alienation arising from the shared perception of meaningless and repetitive occupations and tasks.

These three dimensions in relation to mental health will be explored, illustrated by ordinary encounters from my life.

In the post office

Until recently, I lived and worked in the same locality; so when I see a person I recognise I am not sure where I know the person from. I was waiting in the local post office when I noticed two men in front of me, one with a pension book and the other man who I immediately recognised but could not place. He was tall, wore a broad rimmed hat and had dark hair curling over his shoulders. I knew when he turned towards me that he would be wearing reflective sunglasses and he would have a beard. He was thinner than I remembered. His voice was authoritative: 'Can't understand why things have to be changed. There was nothing wrong before.' I was interested to see what he was complaining about. The man behind the counter had a resigned air. As the man in the hat left, I was overwhelmed by the stale smell of his unwashed clothes. I would not choose to sit next to him on a train for an hour. And this set me thinking about exclusion. How realistic is it to expect people with mental health problems to become integrated into the community? To what extent can I live peacefully alongside someone who does not wash their clothes and argues in post offices?

The conversation in the post office resumed and the man with the pension book spoke about the man in the hat. It seemed that he had been questioning the need for a receipt, 'more bits of paper', and the pension man could not understand his ungratefulness or his bad mood. What was wrong with a scrap of paper? It could be useful, if something went wrong. When something goes wrong, for me, it is inevitably an effort to locate that crucial scrap of paper. And I could see that, for all of us, this episode meant different things. The scrap of paper, for the man in the hat, may have been another burden or another representation of officialdom. The man with the pension book was interested in his reaction, but incredulous. The man behind the counter was resigned and I was thinking about my research.

Critiquing the concept of occupational alienation

It is possible to trace alienation through this experience, linked with the stale smelling clothes, scraps of paper and each of our responses. However, in relation to alienation, it has to be questioned whether the occupational label is useful or distracting. It could be argued that alienation is an emotional state, not related to what people do. Understandings from psychiatry support a concept of alienation being a state of mind; for example, persons with psychosis interpreting their experience in a way not widely shared (Pilgrim, 2005). These persons then become alienated from others, because they have a different view of their experience, or they are alienated from themselves, because their interpretation is at odds with reality or the accepted view of their experience. In contrast, Laing (1967) proposed that alienation is a universal human experience.

Two aspects of alienation deserve further exploration. The first is alienation in a social sense. People can be alienated from others because they see their experience in a different way. Thus, alienation is seen as an alternative to belonging and relates to social inclusion, which promotes belonging as a means of promoting mental health (Bryant *et al.*, 2004). The second aspect of alienation relates to creativity. Returning to the man in the hat, if he was someone who had experienced delusional beliefs about his social status he perceived that this belief was not shared by others, he might feel socially alienated. His interactions could become aggressive and negative, his isolation leading him to neglect those self-care occupations, which would facilitate his belonging. He would be driven to live and do things in different ways because of his sense of a gap between what he wanted and what he was experiencing. He would have to create new possibilities to survive. Beyond mental illness, Lacan's theories of creativity and alienation support this concept (Stavrakakis, 2002). Creative acts arise from an internal sense of alienation, the gap between what is desired and what is actually experienced. A deeper analysis has been offered by Mann (2001).

Similarly, Wilcock's (1998) theory suggested that occupational alienation was signified by a split between the things we have to do and the things we desire to do. She believed that occupational alienation was a key determinant of ill-health, associated with industrialisation. She used a Marxist understanding of alienation (Wilcock, 1998, 2006). Marx (1975) wrote extensively about alienation, linked with the dehumanising effects of industrial production. His analysis of alienation recognised three forms: of the individual from the products of his or her work, from the process of the work and from others. Occupational alienation derives from this. If the products of an individual's activities do not directly meet his or her personal needs, or directly meet the needs of another person known to the originator, the individual is engaged in doing something that is not directly meaningful, and yet he or she continues to do this to live. Thus, the individual is alienated from the process of the occupation as well as from its product. Finally, the individual is alienated from others, being viewed by others in terms of their role in the process of production. Marx's utopian vision to overcome alienation involves human needs being met through a direct transaction between one person and another, meeting needs without the alienating intermediary of money.

So occupational alienation can be seen as a human response when meanings change and occupational forms shift, facilitating the emergence of new meanings and ways of doing. As such it is a significant concept for advancing practice in mental health, where this process is ongoing, as people engage with their problems, avoid them, succumb to them and recover from them. New meanings and ways of doing, or occupational forms, emerge and indicate recovery or relapse.

Efforts to facilitate this process can be seen as overcoming occupational alienation. Setting up opportunities for individuals to create meaningful ways of doing things for themselves may reduce occupational and social alienation, increasing their sense of belonging in the wider social context. Social inclusion is a dynamic process of negotiation between individuals and society, not an outcome in itself. Recognising the shifting meanings applied by the individual and society means that occupational alienation is an intrinsic part of the process of creating new possibilities for belonging. For example, Aggett and Goldberg (2005) describe the group of people they worked with as pervasively alienated, being isolated, inaccessible, invisible, antagonistic and living a rigidly patterned lifestyle. They avoided contact with mental health services, only emerging when symptoms became uncontrollable or housing issues arose. Their sense of alienation often extended to the staff of community mental health teams, preventing creative approaches being developed (Aggett & Goldberg, 2005). A starting point for developing meaningful contact was concerned with the occupational form: doing everyday occupations predictably and in a way with which the service user found meaningful was essential.

Bryant *et al.* (2004) suggested three dimensions of occupational alienation, using the metaphor of living in a glasshouse, which places a barrier between the individual and society. This blocks a sense of belonging, being alienated from others (interpersonal). Vulnerability, represented by the glasshouse, limits the occupations that the person can engage in (occupational). This in turn impacts on the person's sense of self, causing a sense of alienation (intrapersonal). This is illustrated in Figure 7.1.

In the hardware shop

Returning to the man described earlier, I often see him locally but rarely in town. In a crowded shop where the layout had recently changed, I was disorientated; it took me a few minutes to work out where to pay for my purchase. My confusion was compounded by the presence of this man. His appearance was similar but now he wore a long black raincoat. On this occasion his clothes did not smell. He was in the queue behind another man who was being served, and he did not appear to have a purchase to pay for. So I smiled and asked, 'Are you queuing to be served?' He muttered, 'No, no, I'm not queuing.' He walked away as the other man had completed his transaction. They greeted each other and walked out of the shop together. Who was this second man? A friend, partner or support worker?

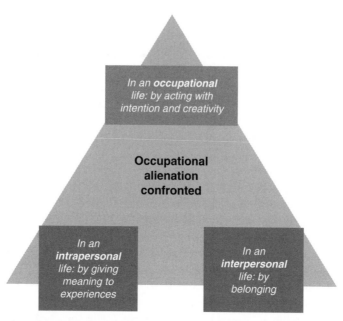

Figure 7.1 Vulnerability, represented by the glasshouse, limits the occupations that the person can engage in (occupational alienation confirmed). This in turn impacts on the person's sense of self, causing a sense of alienation (intrapersonal).

Occupational alienation explored

It was not possible to tell the nature of the relationship between those two men, but their joint activity suggested that there was a sense of belonging and equality in their shared occupation of shopping. Occupational alienation can be overcome by a shift or transformation in one of the three dimensions previously identified: intrapersonal, occupational or interpersonal. The shift perceived here, that the man, previously viewed as isolated and excluded, was engaged in a relationship, could suggest that he had acknowledged his alienation and sought a link with another person. This would have required him to act with intention, risking rejection or rejection. However, if the second man was a support worker, paid to make links, the situation would be different. Neither man would have necessarily chosen to engage with the other. Nevertheless, the situation offered an opportunity to make a link, engage in meaningful occupation and transform the meanings they ascribed to their shared experiences. Negotiating this process unfolds in each therapeutic encounter. If there is no opportunity to find a shared, meaningful dimension to the occupations they do together, then occupational alienation may be the consequence. When occupations are not meaningful, people can be considered to be occupationally alienated. This may drive them to transform intrapersonal and interpersonal meanings in the process of doing. If opportunities to be creative or initiate meaningful occupations are denied or deprived by external forces, this too leads to occupational alienation. Equally, if the occupations deny opportunities to renew and transform a sense of identity or meaning, associated with occupational imbalance, again this leads to occupational alienation.

It is suggested that these aspects are not hierarchical or linear; they evolve and merge. The social dimension of occupation illustrates this. Occupational alienation can be ameliorated by people working or doing things together for a shared purpose. This demands that they have a sense of belonging and acceptance in their group. As meanings shift within and beyond the group, the individual's sense of alienation changes. People generate new ways of doing things, or new things to do, and renegotiate the meaning of these things with others. As such, alienation is intrinsic with occupation, a shared experience and at best, a transitory state.

The practice of occupational therapy creates these shared experiences though groups and creative activities. By doing something in a different way, or doing something different, it is possible to discover new meanings. The beauty of creative activities in occupational therapy is that the created object is often visible to others and so facilitates belonging. Overcoming occupational alienation involves attending to the meanings given to occupations, giving priority to creative occupations and new ways of doing old things, and placing it all in a social context which fosters relationships rather than conflict.

The usefulness of the concept of occupational alienation has been suggested, and the remainder of the chapter will be concerned with exploring this in relation to community mental health and day services in particular. Key issues relating to occupational alienation are meaninglessness and isolation as perceived by the individual and by others, and the lack of opportunity to be creative or control occupations and tasks. These issues relate strongly to current themes in community mental health care, especially social exclusion, social networking and service user involvement.

Social inclusion and social exclusion

Alienation may be associated with those people considered to be socially excluded, for whatever reason. Mental illness is recognised as both a consequence and cause of social exclusion. In 2004, the Social Exclusion Unit's report on mental health included a section on mental health day services (Office of the Deputy Prime Minister, 2004). It was recognised that social exclusion can apply to people or places; so being in a particular place may prevent inclusion as much as who a person is. This aspect is very important in relation to the location of day services, which were seen as a gateway to other community resources, such as paid employment. However, location cannot be regarded as the sole cause of social exclusion. In relation to day services, this implies that a sophisticated understanding of social exclusion is required.

Byrne (2005) suggests that since 1997 the UK government has initiated and developed many policies working for social *inclusion*, viewed as enabling all to participate in social and cultural life, primarily through the generation of wealth from paid employment (Barry & Hallett, 1998). In contrast, the concept of social *exclusion* can create images of people as victims stuck in situations by their own misfortune. Byrne (2005) proposed that a 'weak' sense of social exclusion drives UK policy, changing the individual rather than the context to overcome exclusion. His critique of the Social Exclusion Unit is centred on the failure to ask who is doing the excluding. In terms of social exclusion and mental illness, it could be argued that this has meant focusing on services to create opportunities for individuals to return to paid employment or take up volunteering. This could be at the expense of other recognised ways of promoting social inclusion, for example, building opportunities for social networking.

Social networks

Social networks are advocated as a positive factor in the report on social exclusion and mental health (Office of the Deputy Prime Minister, 2004). The link between effective social networks and health has been explored in theories of social capital (Field, 2003). In terms of mental health day services, suggesting that social networking is a commodity or part of a package to be offered to service users means misunderstanding the dynamic nature of networks. It is not possible to place a person in a social network; it is something achieved by personal action inspired by a sense of meaning and purpose. Capra (2002) emphasises the difficulty in detecting networks from the outside as they are in a constant state of flux. Social networks continually renew themselves through ongoing dialogue about shared meanings, knowledge, ground rules and identity (Capra, 2002). The boundary of the network is also negotiated, offering opportunities for access from new members, but this depends on whether the perceived purpose of the network resonates with the individuals' ideas, or whether they believe it is possible to negotiate inclusion with other network members. Perceiving the network ground rules may be particularly problematic as they are often tacit (Capra, 2002). Because social networks are primarily based within families, close friendships and work setting, accessing them may be difficult. From the outside, the meanings and purposes of the occupations associated with the network may not be perceptible.

Social networks are seen as potential source of support but that is not always their primary purpose. Current mental health policy emphasises the benefits of employment and social networks for recovery, yet issues of support for people with a long-term need for services are not directly addressed. It is possible that social networks are viewed as being synonymous with support networks, but the informal, inaccessible and evolving nature of social networks raise difficulties for those who have already found informal networks insufficient in their recovery process. Repper and Perkins (2003) recognise the need to support the maintenance of relationships, not just for the individual service user, but also for others in their networks. In relation to alienation, social and support networks are associated with a sense of belonging, and so efforts to sustain relationships should impact on a sense of alienation. However, these efforts have to be meaningful to service users and those who support them, and this can only be gauged by effectively involving service users not only in their own journeys within services, but also in service development.

Service user involvement

Involving users in service evaluation and development has been advocated by the National Service Framework for Mental Health (Department of Health, 1999) in response to the dual drivers of a growing user movement and of a political push to improve the quality of services. Service users have sought to influence services and providers are required to listen to them. Barnes and Bowl (2001) and Beresford (2005) distinguish between the user movement and service user involvement in services development and research. Conflicts may arise from the cultural differences between formal, statutory bureaucracies and often informal small-scale user groups. Beresford and Wilson (1998) suggest that redefining the location of expertise is an important first step to involve users to challenge the established status of professionals or independent experts. Boardman (2005) claims that this has been successful to some extent, but has raised new issues, especially for staff who are required to balance being responsive to user perspectives and being responsible for controlling limited resources and risk management. Overcoming these barriers to involvement requires a shift in perspective on equality, valuing everyone's presence and contribution and fostering a sense of ownership by sharing control of the process (Beresford & Wilson, 1998; Beresford, 2005). Assigning equal status to people and events during this process requires continuous negotiation and reflection.

The process of involving services users also involves meaningful occupations, because it is only when people are doing something that their level of participation can be perceived. Understanding the development and evaluation of services from an occupational perspective requires analysis of all the tasks, skills and activities available (Molineux, 2004). Recognition of these components provides opportunities for participation in change and meaningful inclusion. Conversely, when it becomes apparent that service users are not engaging with these opportunities, the concept of occupational alienation can inform dialogue.

Community care and day services

Social exclusion, social networking and service user involvement have a particular focus in day services. Day services have been primarily occupation-focused, concentrating on meaningful time use and/or acquisition of skills for participation in the community (Bender & Pilling, 1985; Catty et al., 2001; Davis et al., 2004; Bryant et al., 2005) and/or therapy/training, including vocational and social skills (Yurkovitch, 1999). The history of mental health services emphasises institutional care, rather than community care (Bartlett & Wright, 1999). The shift from hospital to community services occurred over several decades: initiatives in community care predated the NHS with the first day hospitals being established in 1946

(Boardman, 2005). Occupational therapists became involved; Wilcock (2002) cited a 1963 example of a day programme created by an occupational therapist. The programme shifted between treating people with psychological interventions as day patients and giving them something meaningful to do, somewhere to go and a structure for their day. With an occupational perspective, these two aspects are not mutually exclusive. However, current service provision emphasises individual interventions to facilitate recovery and individual occupational interventions within the community to facilitate inclusion. This emphasis ignores the possibility that occupational interventions incorporate psychological benefits. Equally, the emphasis on individual interventions ignores the social context for recovery, especially in terms of shared experience and empowerment and the resource implications for addressing needs primarily on an individual basis.

Two issues emerged from my experience in community mental health day services in the early 1990s. First, institutional care was confused with care in specific buildings, triggering the idea that if you take away the building, you will prevent institutionalisation. Second, that institutional care was associated with grouping people together according to need. It was believed that if these groups were dispersed, institutionalisation care would be avoided. This ignored understandings of institutionalisation as a cultural and social process, related to the use and abuse of power, regardless of buildings (Foster, 1998). In addition, it is a way of using resources most effectively to meet a shared need, and will arise wherever this need is perceived to streamline social interaction and settle power relations. In this understanding of institutionalisation, the proposed 'gateway' role of day services (Office of the Deputy Prime Minister, 2004) will inevitably be associated with efforts to meet shared needs. The needs that are recognised and engaged with will depend on how power is distributed between service users and service providers.

Davis *et al.* (2004) placed day services in a wider context in which community mental health services were split and increasingly focused on specific and apparently separate tasks. This focus was claimed to have benefits for service users, but only so long as services were integrated with each other. Day services took on a bridge-builder role, facilitating access to other mental health services and mainstream community resources. It was possible to sustain both a safe space and a link to other services. However, the bridge-builder role is challenged by a conceptualisation associated with social capital. Whilst bridge-building enables people to develop, bonding is also required to enable people to survive (Almedom, 2005). Favouring the development of people over and above their survival, for example, by giving priority to employment initiatives within day services, could have a negative impact on service users, causing them to become occupationally alienated. Bonding is associated with a sense of belonging.

The particular challenge of current times has been how to balance the rise in professional power, underpinned by legislation in health and social care, with the informality and ambiguity required for community living (Bartlett & Wright, 1999). Tomlinson (1991, p. 163) noted that 'The aloneness in the community of a significant proportion of service recipients, and their relative lack of opportunity for giving and receiving mutual support', with professional efforts to facilitate integration failing. It could be argued that non-institutional care, in its benign sense, is not achievable as some shared needs have to be met on a collective or group basis. Leighton (2003) challenges the emphasis on individualised approaches, detailing the varied collective approaches to mental health care and their benefits. Organisational control of mental health services remains as strong as ever (Townsend, 1998). At the service provision level, in the UK, whilst there is much emphasis on person-centred care and informal settings for contact, this is strongly countered by procedural constraints associated with risk management, the Care Programme Approach and resource management policies. So users may have contact with services in non-institutional places, but the nature, process and possible outcomes of that contact will be bound by institutional codes of practice and procedures.

One of the beliefs pervading contemporary community day services is that individuals will return to the community. For many, this might mean resuming the life they led prior to becoming ill. For others, this is a less clear concept. Cleaver (2001) argues that the community is often viewed as a single body with clear geographical boundaries, usually convergent with institutional boundaries. This denies the differentiated nature of communities. Even communities that seem close-knit may struggle to accommodate the needs of all their members all of time. In relation to mental health, day services idealisation of the community has a great influence on how services are promoted and valued.

However, difficulties remain with buildings and the concept of social inclusion. Cheetham and Fuller (1998) suggest that a particular location will bring excluded people together, providing opportunities and a safe place to be. However, the building itself may be a symbol of exclusion in itself, as mental-health-associated buildings often are, adding to the sense of exclusion. Repper and Perkins (2003) suggest that the stigma associated with attendance at a day centre cannot be underestimated.

From an occupational perspective, the function of an environment is indicated by more than the bricks of the physical building; the social, cultural and institutional aspects will interface with the people who use it (Canadian Association of Occupational Therapists, 1997). The impact of the environment is given a political dimension by Townsend and Wilcock (2004) who explored the interconnectedness of human occupation through the concept of occupational justice. Whilst there are similarities with social justice, the focus on the right to participate in meaningful occupation incorporates a perceived responsibility at individual level as well as organisational level. The recognition of occupational justice has forced occupational therapists, a self-proclaimed apolitical profession, to acknowledge the political nature of occupation, precipitating explorations of how power is expressed through what we do (Kronenberg *et al.*, 2004).

There is an emphasis on individual difference in configuration of occupations within occupational justice (Townsend & Wilcock, 2004). Alongside this is an embedded recognition of unpaid occupations as being of equivalent value to society to paid occupations, thus challenging the prevailing cultural, political and institutional focus on paid occupations as a means of achieving a fair and just society.

Occupational justice as conceptualised by Townsend and Wilcock (2004) recognises that all health-promoting occupations underpin not only the health of individuals but also society as a whole.

Summary

This chapter has explored occupational alienation, a complex concept arising from barriers to opportunities to act creatively and with intention, in a meaningful way at personal and social level. These issues have been explored in relation to mental health day services. Occupational alienation is a useful concept to inform the emphasis of day services, shifting focus to the need for people to belong to services, to have opportunities for meaningful and creative occupations and to have space to reflect on the personal and social meanings that evolve and emerge. The concept is particularly relevant at the current time, when every element of service delivery is translated into targets and thus is alienated from the human dimension of the staff and service users who work together in day services. As a result, creative approaches are stifled, belonging is discouraged and pressures are so relentless that reflection on personal and social meanings is deferred. Fostering a sense of belonging within a culture of reflection and creative action counterbalances occupational alienation: this applies to all involved, service users, staff and everyone else.

Questioning your Practice

1. In your work setting can you identify people who are alienated and identify the intrapersonal, interpersonal and occupational dimensions of their alienation?
2. Which therapeutic strategies used in your setting may contribute to alienation?
3. How could these strategies be adapted to diminish alienation?

References

Aggett P, Goldberg D (2005) Pervasive alienation: on seeing the invisible, meeting the inaccessible and engaging 'lost to contact' clients with major mental illness. *Journal of Interprofessional Care, 19(2)*, 83–92.

Almedom A (2005) Social capital and mental health: an interdisciplinary review of primary evidence. *Social Science & Medicine, 61(5)*, 943–964.

Barnes M, Bowl R (2001) *Taking Over the Asylum*. Basingstoke: Palgrave.

Barry M, Hallett C (eds) (1998) *Social Exclusion and Social Work*. Lyme Regis: Russell House Publishing Ltd.

Bartlett P, Wright D (1999) Community care and its antecedents. In: P Bartlett, D Wright (eds) *Outside the Walls of the Asylum. The History of Care in the Community 1750–2000*. London: The Athlone Press, 1–19.

Bender M, Pilling S (1985) A study of variables associated with under-attendance at a psychiatric day hospital. *Psychological Medicine, 15(2),* 395–401.

Beresford P (2005) Social approaches to madness and distress: user perspectives and user knowledges. In: J Tew (ed.) *Social Perspectives in Mental Health.* London: Jessica Kingsley, 13–31.

Beresford P, Wilson A (1998) Challenging the contradiction of exclusive debate. In: M Barry, C Hallett, (eds) (1998) *Social Exclusion and Social Work.* Lyme Regis: Russell House Publishing Ltd.

Boardman J (2005) New services for old – an overview of mental health policy. In: A Bell, P Lindley, (eds) *Beyond the water towers.* London: Sainsbury Centre for Mental Health, 27–36.

Brewer P, Gadsen V, Scrimshaw K (1994) The community group network in mental health: a model for social support and community integration. *British Journal of Occupational Therapy, 57(12),* 467–470.

Bryant W (1991) Creative groupwork and the elderly mentally ill: a development of sensory integration therapy. *British Journal of Occupational Therapy, 54(5),* 187–192.

Bryant W (1995) The Social Contact Group: an example of long term group work in community mental health. *British Journal of Occupational Therapy, 58(5), 214-18.*

Bryant W, Craik C, McKay E (2004) Living in a glass house: exploring occupational alienation. *Canadian Journal of Occupational Therapy, 5(71),* 282–289.

Bryant W, Craik C, McKay EA (2005) Perspectives of day and accommodation services for people with enduring mental illness. *Journal of Mental Health, 14(2),* 109–120.

Byrne D (2005) *Social Exclusion.* (2nd edn). Maidenhead: Open University Press.

Canadian Association of Occupational Therapists (1997) *Enabling Occupation: An Occupational Therapy perspective.* Ottawa: Canadian Association of Occupational Therapists.

Capra F (2002) *The Hidden Connections.* London: Flamingo.

Catty J, Burns T, Comas A (2001) Day centres for severe mental illness. *Cochrane Database of Systematic Reviews,* 2001 *(2),* http://www.mrw.interscience.wiley.com/cochrane/clsysrev/articles/re10001/CD001710/frame.html.

Cheetham J, Fuller R (1998) Social exclusion and social work: policy, practice and research. In: M Barry, C Hallett (eds) *Social Exclusion and Social Work.* Lyme Regis: Russell House Publishing Ltd.

Cleaver F (2001) Institutions, agency and the limitations of participatory approaches to development. In: B Cooke, U Korthari (eds) *Participation: The New Tyranny?* London: Zed Books, 36–55.

Davis F, Alder S, Jones P (2004) Day services modernisation and social inclusion. *A Life in the Day, 8(3),* 18–24.

Department of Health (1999) *National Service Framework for Mental Health, Executive Summary.* London: The Stationery Office.

Field (2003) *Social Capital.* London: Routledge.

Foster A (1998) Thinking about risk. In: A Foster, V Roberts (eds) *Managing Mental Health in the Community, Chaos and containment.* London: Routledge, pp. 84–94.

Jung C, Winston R, Winston C (1995) *Memories, Dreams, Reflections.* London: Fontana.

Kronenberg F, Simo Algado S, Pollard N (2004) *Occupational Therapy without Borders, Learning from the Spirit of Survivors.* Oxford: Churchill Livingstone.

Laing R (1967) *The Politics of Experience.* Harmondsworth: Penguin Books Ltd.

Leighton K (2003) A social conflict analysis of collective mental health care: past, present and future. *Journal of Mental Health, 12(5),* 475–488.

Mann S (2001) Alternative perspectives on the student experience: alienation and engagement. *Studies in Higher Education, 26(1),* 7–19.

Marx K (1975) *Early Writings*. Harmondsworth: Penguin Books.

Molineux M (ed) (2004) *Occupation for Occupational Therapists*. Oxford: Blackwell Publishing Ltd.

Office of the Deputy Prime Minister (2004) *Mental Health and Social Exclusion, Social Exclusion Unit Report Summary*. London: Office of the Deputy Prime Minister.

Pilgrim D (2005) *Key Concepts in Mental Health*. London: Sage Publications.

Repper J, Perkins R (2003) *Social Inclusion and Recovery*. Edinburgh: Balliere Tindall.

Stavrakakis Y(2002) Creativity and its limits: encounters with social constructionism and the political in Castoriadis and Lacan. *Constellations, 9(4)*, 522–539.

Tomlinson D (1991) *Utopia, Community Care and the Retreat from the Asylums*. Milton Keynes: Open University Press.

Townsend E (1998) *Good Intentions Overruled: A Critique of Empowerment in the Routine Organisation of Mental Health Services*. Toronto: University of Toronto Press.

Townsend E, Wilcock A (2004) Occupational justice. In: C Christiansen, E Townsend (eds) *Introduction to Occupation*. New Jersey: Prentice Hall, pp. 243–273.

Wilcock A (1998) *An Occupational Perspective of Health*. New Jersey: Slack Inc.

Wilcock A (2002) *Occupation for Health. Volume 2: A Journey from Prescription to Self Health*. London: College of Occupational Therapists, 314–316.

Wilcock A (2006) *An Occupational Perspective of Health* (2nd edn). New Jersey: Slack Inc.

Yerxa E (2000) Confessions of an occupational therapist who became a detective. *British Journal of Occupational Therapy, 63(5)*, 192–199.

Yurkovich E, Smyer T, Dean L (1999) Maintaining health: proactive client-oriented community day treatment centres for the chronic mentally ill. *Journal of Psychiatric and Mental Health Nursing, 6(1)*, 61–69.

Zemke R, Clark F (eds) (1996) *Occupational Science. The Evolving Discipline*. Philadelphia: F A Davis Company.

8 Strengths and challenges to practice
Reconciling occupational justice issues as a prerequisite to mental health recovery

Karen L. Rebeiro Gruhl

Personal narrative

I am an occupational therapist who practises in northeastern Ontario in Canada. It covers 1 million km^2 and constitutes 90% of the surface area of Ontario, although it has only 5% of the population. It is economically, politically, geographically and socially different from the rest of the province. The district where I work has large distances between cities and towns, severe winter weather and the associated travelling hazards and high unemployment rates and fewer people completing high-school. I have worked in a non-typical practice for the past 20 years. Whether this is non-typical by intention, opportunity or otherwise is hard to say. This is just how it evolved or unfolded in my life. What is unique about my story are the necessary partnerships that I have negotiated with mental health consumers to conduct research and to provide care in my region. This remains both a strength and challenge of my practice. Additionally challenging have been my ongoing attempts to maintain a research and publication profile despite this aspect of my work being removed 3 years ago when I was requested to return to a full-time clinical position. It was difficult to go back, although understandably necessary, given the current shortages of occupational therapists in my region. It is equally daunting to move forward in my pursuit of a PhD, juggling full-time work and a family, in addition to book projects and publications. But this is where I sit as I write this chapter.

I graduated in 1985. I did not intend to work in mental health but, instead, in some rather acute, dramatic and terribly exciting area of practice, like burns or splinting hand injuries (though, truth be told, I was not good in either of those areas). It happened that the only position available when I graduated was in mental health, and likewise, when I relocated to Northern Ontario in 1987, mental health was the position that was immediately available. This was not meant to happen. I really had no interest in mental health 20 years ago. The same cannot be said today.

I have always found mental health practice to be equally exhilarating and frustrating, but I have always been slightly embarrassed by some past practices of the profession, resulting in a lack of understanding, valuing and respect attributed to occupational therapy in mental health. Given that, I always strived to do a good job on behalf of my profession, but something was always missing for me.

The focus of my practice has been to make a difference, albeit a small one, in the lives of my clients. There have been many times throughout these 20 years when I have questioned whether I was making that difference, or for that matter, whether any one really cared whether an occupational therapist was involved in their client's care. My earlier career years, like many of my classmates and colleagues, were tainted by self-doubt about roles, about the contribution of occupational therapy, especially in typically underserviced areas. I responded to this role confusion in a typical occupational therapy way – I became useful and expanded my boundaries to include just about everything that I perceived to be missing – my role became to fill in the gaps.

I quickly learn that many of the 'recipes' that I had been taught in my undergraduate education were being conducted by assistants or other health professionals, even if the programme or groups had been developed by occupational therapists. The reality was that occupational therapists did not remain in the North for very long. New graduates came North on incentive bursaries and, once their time commitment expired, would typically return to southern Ontario. This was very frustrating for me and others who chose to stay in the North and who did not receive a financial incentive to do so. There were two main reasons for this. First, the health community in which I practised had limited experience of the profession – usually a new graduate who did not fully appreciate what an occupational therapist could offer the health care system. Second, as an occupational therapist, I continually struggled to define a unique and visible professional role for myself. I became tired of explaining what an occupational therapist did, or could do, and, worse, of being dictated to, by what the team thought an occupational therapist should do or had done in the past.

So for the first 10 years in northern Ontario, I worked hard and yet felt unsatisfied. I was receiving positive feedback from others and helping clients in a variety of ways; however, it would be difficult to defend what I did as occupational therapist. In truth, in 1994 I did not know what authentic occupational therapy was or whether, in fact, there was such a thing!

Subsequently, one of the wisest things I did was to return to graduate school. I needed to learn how to better describe what I did, how to influence clinical care and services and to learn research skills and strategies. This would assist me to provide the kind of evidence that health care systems required and which I felt ill prepared to provide at that time. In 1995, I made the decision to go to graduate school to learn how to do research so that I could provide evidence for what I was doing, prove my worth as an occupational therapist or attempt to change the system. Or, perhaps, I could use research as a way to figure out this frustrating system!

The stories of individual clients within the system began to emerge. Their lack of participation in the processes of care and the paucity of opportunities to be involved in 'occupation-based' therapy or occupation as a goal in community became highlighted through research. I realised, then, how frustrated clients were with the mental health system and, remarkably, how the clients' frustration was similar to my own as an occupational therapist working in an under-resourced region.

Although I did not necessarily realise it at the time, it became increasingly obvious to me that consumers were likely the best group to work with, to conduct research with and to attempt to change the system with.

Through research, I began to learn how clients viewed therapy and these lessons were sometimes painful (Rebeiro, 2000). I began to learn how clients experienced the mental health system in the North (Rebeiro, 1999); and I began to learn about how clients had many good ideas about what needed to change and how to go about this process (Rebeiro *et al.*, 2001). The clients and I were both working hard, seemingly getting nowhere and were both equally frustrated! Instead of viewing clients through the lens of client–therapist relationships, I learnt about the mental health system through the lens of the recipient of care, and subsequently gained a better appreciation of what it was like to be an individual client navigating through the mental health system. For me, the entire process was actually a fairly circuitous and lengthy route to gain a straightforward position in empathy. By asking questions, observing and listening, I was better able to learn about the system that I worked in from the very individuals I was paid to help. It was a humbling experience and also life altering with respect to how I would thereafter practise as an occupational therapist and how I would view occupational therapy's role within the system. I believe that one cannot go back once one is in touch with this client-centred perspective. It naturally opens up a different view, as the way you approach your work helps to define what you are prepared to do, or not, within the future health-care system.

For example, a research study designed to learn more about how mental health consumers spend their time on a daily basis, specifically how they approached their search for meaningful occupation within the community, yielded several insights (Rebeiro, 1999). Although my practice had required that I connect and work with community agencies, I was in reality still fairly hospital-bound. By looking at client movement and perspectives beyond my typical environment, I was able to learn about the effectiveness of therapy in a hospital setting and whether it helped clients to successfully bridge their occupational performance into the community. These gradual insights have helped me to change my thinking of the mental health system and of the importance of the environment (Rebeiro, 2003; Strong & Rebeiro, 2003). An important aspect of my research is that I remain, first and foremost, a clinical occupational therapist and all of my research either stems from clinical practice or irritants, or flows back into the work that I do with clients. Research has helped me to be less egocentric or profession-focused and more client-centred. Similarly, it has also assisted me to forge long-standing partnerships with a variety of consumer groups and organisations.

Since 1997, I have invested a great deal of energy in the development of an occupation-based collaboration with consumers known as Northern Initiative for Social Action (NISA) (Rebeiro *et al.*, 2001). It is a consumer-run, occupation-based programme of initiatives developed from collaborative research that aimed to address the paucity of occupational opportunity in my area (see http:// www.nisa.on.ca). I used to work closely with this group, but they are now self-sufficient and I now attend a half day each week.

I have also attempted to explore and better understand the many systemic issues regarding the provision of mental health services, in particular occupation-based interventions in the North, the geographic context in which I live and work (Legault & Rebeiro, 2001; Rebeiro *et al.*, 2001; Wright & Rebeiro, 2003). Many of these small projects were conducted with consumers as research partners.

Currently, I am the sole occupational therapist at a community mental health clinic that provides medication support, intensive case management and rehabilitation for persons with serious mental illness. My roles and responsibilities are divided between some case management responsibilities, consulting to the team, providing assessment and treatment (both individual and group), providing clinical support to NISA programme and staff, and some research/educational responsibilities, including students. It is a juggle to manage, and despite many positive attributes about the clinic, my work in practice remains a frustration. Thus, the only way to reconcile the many conflicts I have about my present and future clinical work was to conduct more research. I enrolled in a PhD programme.

Influences to practice

During graduate school, the work of Ann Wilcock (1993) and her thoughtful dialogue on the human need for occupation was influential. Her work provided a basis for reflection on practice, the need for occupation, in particular for those individuals often denied such experiences, such as mental health consumers. Additionally, Wilcock's work gave the grounding to look deeper into the meaning and experience of occupational engagement for mental health consumers in research (Rebeiro, 1999; Rebeiro & Allen, 1998; Rebeiro & Cook, 1999). These initial research projects dovetailed into a further series of studies geared to better understand the phenomenon of occupational engagement, its lived experience and its value to mental health consumers (Legault & Rebeiro, 2001; Rebeiro, 1999; Rebeiro *et al.*, 2001; Wright & Rebeiro, 2003). These projects and the rationale behind them have been previously shared in J. V. Cook's qualitative textbook, *Qualitative Research in Occupational Therapy* (2001) and more recently in Hammell and Carpenter's (2003), *Qualitative Research in Evidence-Based Rehabilitation*.

Townsend's (1993, 1998, 2003) ideas on empowerment, on a social vision for the profession and on how the good intentions of occupational therapy in mental health are often submerged or overruled by more dominant forces and systems have been significant. The idea of power, its influence in mental health practice, especially in the realm of a primarily women-dominated profession, although not surprising were disturbing. Sadly, Townsend's ethnography of mental health and occupational therapy practice in eastern Canada resonated with my practice in northern Ontario. Townsend's research convinced me that I needed to pay closer attention to power relations and later to issues of justice.

The ongoing dialogue on occupational justice generated by Townsend and Wilcock (2004) was very instrumental in shaping thoughts and ideas on implementing a recovery-based mental health system in an occupationally deprived region such as north-eastern Ontario. The idea of providing opportunities (a sharing of resources), as opposed to perceiving that more money or professional staff would be required to address the deprivation, began to germinate. The issues of justice provided a more reasonable or accurate explanation of why mental health consumers did not participate more fully in occupation and, through this process of engagement, promote their own recoveries. It seemed that, to do so, occupational opportunity would need to be more of a standard aspect of the multi-disciplinary care process than how it appeared to currently exist. Furthermore, the creation of partnerships with community-based opportunities would need to be fostered to provide choice and opportunity for occupational engagement as an integral component of any recovery-based system of care (MacGillivary & Nelson, 1998; Rebeiro, Nov 2002; Rebeiro, 2004).

So I began an attempt to understand why there were (and are) so few occupational opportunities for therapy and for recovery-based work in the North-east despite policy documents that suggest that occupation may be one of the components of long-term management of mental illness (Ministry of Health [MOH], 2001) and an integral component of an individual's recovery. Mental health consumers in north-eastern Ontario continue to lack occupation in practice and in the community. Many consumers do not find the community inclusive or welcoming to begin with, and the social exclusion they experience often results in occupational marginalisation by virtue of stigma (Rebeiro, 1999). Collectively, occupational alienation, deprivation and marginalisation appeared to provide the best plausible explanation for the recovery of persons with mental illness in this area. This insight prompted further research questions:

1. Is the provision of occupational opportunity an integral aspect of the recovery-oriented services offered by the multi-disciplinary team in mental health care in rural and northern Ontario?
2. If yes, how does the team go about providing occupation-based 'therapy' in the absence of an occupational therapist?
3. If yes, and in the absence of readily available occupational opportunity, does the multi-disciplinary team seek out community partnerships to establish occupational opportunity and/or create occupational opportunity in their clients' community?
4. If no, are the constructs of occupational justice (alienation, deprivation, marginalisation) known and relevant constructs. If so, do these constructs help to serve as real or perceived barriers to consumers' pursuit of and/or participation in occupational opportunities in rural and northern Ontario?

These preliminary ideas, a few small research projects conducted with consumers as partners, and a regional mental health system that remains to date quite medically oriented, underfunded and fragmented, are the driving forces for this work. Equally they create challenges and opportunities in attempting to provide recovery-oriented care as an occupational therapist.

These provide the inspiration for the reflections in this chapter; that seeks to better understand recovery as a systemic construct; the pragmatics of implementing a recovery-based system in a vast, rural, geographic region; and specifically, understanding the characteristics of a recovery attitude. Such an attitude seems important to the recruitment and education of providers, many of the stated barriers to recovery for these people may stem from a variety of injustices of an occupational nature.

Many people did not have the opportunity or the means to engage in occupation, and therefore they do not experience the transformative benefits of engaging in occupation that appeared so important to one's sense of self, one's social identity and mental health recovery (Deegan, 1988; Rebeiro & Cook, 1999; MOH, 2001; Gould *et al.*, 2005; Rebeiro Gruhl, 2006a). Furthermore, engagement in occupation was not necessarily recognised as being important at the provider level and within the multi-disciplinary team; it was not incorporated into goals or care plans, nor was the creation of occupational opportunities in either urban or rural communities a priority, despite high unemployment rates for persons with a disability throughout the region (Nangia *et al.*, 2005).

While not yet formally recognised by the government, this dialogue remains important for many people who are isolated by geography, who continue to be systematically denied opportunities for participation in meaningful and society-valued occupation and who, by lack of experience in and/or exposure to the benefits of participation in occupation, remain alienated from society and, therefore, limited in their capacity to contribute to society and to their own personal recovery journeys. The system may not be ready for this paradigm shift. It is likened to a Kuhnian revolution, and we are currently in the midst of the crisis (Kuhn, 1970).

Reconciling occupational justice issues as a prerequisite to mental health recovery

A qualitative research study aimed to identify the enablers and barriers to recovery from both provider and consumer perspectives, within a large geographic area of north-eastern Ontario (Rebeiro Gruhl, 2006a). This study consisted of three phases: Phase 1 was the survey questionnaire; Phase 2 was the three focus groups that aimed to explore the information and insights generated by survey responses; Phase 3 involved the final two focus groups to explore the recovery attitude. In total, 150 people from 17 distinct communities across the region participated in either survey or focus groups. The constant comparative method of data analysis (Glaser & Strauss, 1967) led to the identification of five enablers or transitional markers to one's recovery path, as well as highlighted the importance of hope and of a 'recovery attitude' to promoting recovery (Figure 8.1).

Interestingly, this research has additionally highlighted many of the occupational injustices that plague mental health consumers in the region and which may be a barrier to their individual recoveries. Despite the research participants' repeated statements regarding the importance of having varied, meaningful and socially relevant opportunities to participate in as an integral aspect of their recovery, few reported such opportunities in their communities. Some of the reasons stated were as a result of the geographic context (weather and distance, culture and climate) of

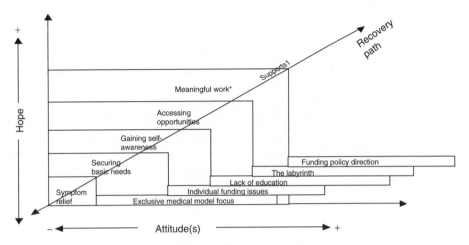

Figure 8.1 The recovery path.

northern Ontario, and some were a result of the structure and composition of the mental health system itself. Participants reported that the opportunities provided to them were largely demeaning, determined by others (versus being client-chosen or client-driven), and were not negotiated with them as a part of, and integral to, their individual recovery processes. The availability of paid work is extremely limited, with equal numbers of disabled and able-bodied persons competing for the same limited number of minimum wage jobs (Statistics Canada, 2001). In the mental health population, studies estimate the rate of unemployment for people with serious mental illness to range from 75% to 89% (Wasylenki *et al.*, 1985). Consequently, there is a need for the creation of occupational opportunity by providers, or collaborative partnerships with community, if occupation is to become a relevant aspect of the individual recovery process and recovery-oriented care.

Figure 8.1 is an attempt to deconstruct and describe the parameters of a recovery-based system of care as articulated by the study participants. It also illustrates why occupation continues to play a lesser role in mental health care in the North-east. Implications for addressing occupational justice and injustices in recovery-based mental health practice are considered (Figure 8.1).

The study's findings and discussion

The participants in Phases 1 and 2 of the study identified five transitional enablers of recovery as well as the preliminary elements of a recovery attitude. As seen in Figure 8.1, these enablers are symptom relief, securing basic needs, gaining self-awareness, accessing opportunities and meaningful work. These enablers are used to structure the remainder of this chapter. Each enabler is hierarchical and builds upon successful resolution of previous stages prior to further progression in one's recovery. Supports were identified as being important to help bridge the barriers in the way of recovery at the various stages, all progress being largely facilitated by the presence of a hopeful attitude in providers. Negative staff attitudes were the most pervasive barrier to an individual's recovery at any stage.

Phase 3 of the study was conducted 5 months later in a different venue and with different participants. This phase of the research consisted of two focus groups, which specifically explored with participants what a recovery attitude would look and feel like. Findings emphasised how clients proceed through recovery and how providers and family members can either help or hinder this process. The findings highlight the systemic change required to realise a recovery vision and further take into consideration the occupational injustices that may well hold the best explanation for limited recoveries in north-eastern Ontario.

Symptom relief

Participants spoke openly about the importance of symptom relief to recovery, often stating that it is difficult, if not impossible, to progress through the various stages if one 'is actively hallucinating' or 'so depressed that they cannot get out of bed'. Participants were clear in stating that relief, not control or cure of symptoms, was the goal in early recovery. The primary role of medication in symptom relief is well established, but clients often spend many years before finding the right medication or gaining a level of self-awareness that they need to take medication. The recovery literature clearly advocates that clients need not be symptom-free (Anthony, 1993, 2000) to be offered programmes and services. The importance of occupational engagement to grounding psychosis in tangible and reality-based processes (Hatchard & Missiuna, 2003), as well as using a variety of occupations to re-engage the mind and body (Gould et al., 2005) have been documented elsewhere. To limit engagement in occupation may serve as a barrier to recovery and may contribute to the initial sense of occupational alienation.

Occupational alienation

According to Townsend and Wilcock (2004), 'occupational alienation is named here as a social condition of injustice, not a psychological state…occupational alienation with prolonged experiences of disconnectedness, isolation, emptiness, lack of a sense of identity, a limited or confined expression of spirit, or a sense of meaninglessness' (p. 80).

Alienation from the opportunity to participate in occupation naturally sets one apart in society. This is further compounded by the marginalisation experienced by mental health consumers because of stigma and poverty and by the deprivation resulting from a lack of funding, choices and opportunities within community either to earn a livelihood or to serve as an aspect of their recovery plan. Being alienated from participation in occupation lends itself to a lack of familiarity or an embodied recognition that participation is important to recovery. Earlier studies demonstrate that an individual's sense of actualisation contributes to a sense of anticipation, or hopefulness, which in turn initiates occupational spin-off. This is a process by which individuals actively seek out other occupational opportunities to sustain their sense of competency and well-being (Rebeiro & Cook, 1999). The recovery research identified that being hopeful was the single most important contributor to progression in one's recovery.

Securing basic needs

The basic needs level encompasses everything from physical and emotional safety to housing and financial support: the necessities of life. Ensuring that the client has an income source, access to medical care including a drug plan, a place to live in and food are important components of recovery-oriented care. Employment also has been shown to have a significant effect on a person's physical, mental and social health. Paid work provides not only money but also a sense of identity and purpose, social contacts and opportunities for personal growth. When people lose these benefits, the results can be devastating to both the health of the individual and that of their family. Unemployed people have a reduced life expectancy and suffer significantly more health problems than people who have a job (Public Health Agency of Canada, 1999). Ensuring that clients have access to and/or opportunity to participate in the economic fabric of life is another aspect of recovery. The research suggests that earlier participation in occupation, especially those involving self-care and community living skills, may expedite attainment of basic needs level of recovery (Gould *et al.*, 2005). The basic needs level is where individuals are likely to first experience occupational marginalisation due to illness, systems or social exclusion.

Occupational marginalisation

According to Townsend and Wilcock (2004, p. 82), 'occupational marginalisation may occur, for instance, when people with disabilities are excluded from employment opportunities, and have few expectations that employment is even possible'. Being marginalised or placed on the outskirts of society is another method by which mental health consumers lose their sense of belonging and perceive being relegated, as one participant said, to the 'useless pile in society' (Rebeiro Gruhl, 2006b). Additionally, occupational marginalisation is fostered by a belief that the mentally ill are too sick to work, or to need to work (Rebeiro, 1999). According to Townsend and Wilcock (2004), 'the argument is that choice and control in what we do to participate in occupations is the basis of our empowerment as humans, and empowerment is a determinant of health for individuals and populations' (p. 82). The recovery study demonstrated that a lack of choice and control creates barriers to one's capacity to participate in occupations in general and employment in particular. This prompts further questions such as: How does employment become addressed in mental health policy and practice? What beliefs and values underscore the decision making of policy? How might occupational therapists, or any member of the interdisciplinary team, foster employment issues at both the practice and policy level, both as a means to recovery and as a matter of justice?

Gaining self-awareness

According to the participants, an individual's capacity to gain self-awareness marks the point of departure between those who move further forward in their recovery from those who do not, who become stuck or reverse into basic needs and symptom relief (Rebeiro Gruhl, 2006a). Indeed, this stage is the clear point of departure between those who are able to meet their basic needs from those who are able to achieve higher level needs. Included in this stage are the issues of moving beyond the system, assuming more responsibility for oneself, wellness and life, and how to manage a serious mental illness and still have a life. This stage is also characterised by internalising hope; that is, people no longer need to look beyond themselves to instil hope. Importantly, the focus of their lives becomes more about what they will do next, future orientated, and less focused on what it has been or on illness-related matters.

Participants stated that part of gaining self-awareness is reconciling to the illness 'stuff' and coming to terms with it, what it means to and for the individual and how to move past it and/or incorporate it into life choices and occupational plans/ goals. According to one survey participant, 'gaining self-awareness involves learning from the illness experience and growing from that experience. The person suffering from mental illness understands the illness and feels whole/accepted/ connected/valued despite the illness. Their worldview, sense of meaning, spiritual context is deepened and strengthened by the mental illness'.

The key barriers identified to gaining self-awareness were individual attitudes and understanding of the possibility of recovery, limited education regarding recovery and how to do it and unsuccessful transition of the earlier stages of symptom relief and securing basic needs. To successfully navigate this stage, the focus-group participants identified the importance of a positive peer role model.

Accessing opportunities

The next stage identified by focus-group participants involved accessing opportunities, such as programmes and services available in one's community. This stage involved navigating a variety of barriers perceived to be present in the larger community, including stigma and the convoluted maze of programmes and services. All participants perceived that the community was complex and not easily navigated and its lack of organisation posed a significant barrier to an individuals' level of participation in community. Further, and according to one participant, 'oftentimes a consumer is expected to seek assistance in the community when they are least able to do so'.

Peer and professional support were deemed to be important to find a way through the community and to making initial contacts with programmes and service opportunities. Movement is often realised once participation in opportunities begins to consolidate a sense of self-confidence and competence and the consumer entertains the idea of exploring work options. When the client is ready for work and few opportunities exist, the injustice of occupational deprivation becomes a reality.

Occupational deprivation

Whiteford (2000) defines deprivation as 'a state of prolonged preclusion from engagement in occupations of necessity and/or meaning due to factors that stand outside the control of the individual' (p. 222). With respect to the recovery study, participants repeatedly stated that 'when there is nothing to do, nothing is what they do'. This 'cycle of do-nothing-ism' (Rebeiro Gruhl, 2006b) perpetuates itself and creates negative routines, habits and occupational patterns (Erlandsson *et al.*, 2004) that are entrenched and difficult to alter when attempting to reintroduce occupational participation into the client's recovery plan.

Focus-group participants spoke of the injustices of limited services, geographic distances to programmes and few or no choices, and that people did not push their own agenda for fear of being discharged with no one left to provide care unless they travelled great distances. The result of geography and limited funding in north-eastern Ontario may contribute to occupational deprivation for many consumers. Again, these findings stimulate further questions: If recovery is limited by occupational deprivation, how do consumers, providers and service agencies address this? How does this impact on equitable access to work?

Meaningful work

Work was identified as the final stage of recovery. The participants spoke of work as an elusive entity. Often they are not offered work – occupational deprivation; told not to work because of stress – occupational alienation; not able to find work in their communities – occupational marginalisation; or offered work that is boring or demeaning – social exclusion. The health benefits to work are well researched in both the physical health and mental health communities. People who work enjoy better physical and mental health and a better quality of life, and, for the mental health population, use less services and hospital bed days than those who are not working (Public Health Agency of Canada, 1999). Likewise, it is widely acknowledged that unemployment is generally associated with negative health outcomes – including diminished mental health and physical well-being (MOH, 2001): 'Employment then is an important determinant for mental and physical health. Yet it remains the case that mental illness can be a tremendous obstacle to an individual's attempts to find and hold employment' (p. 1).

If work is known to promote mental and physical health, quality of life and well-being, and the participants in this study clearly and unanimously identified work as being important to their recovery, why then is work such an 'elusive entity' for mental health consumers in north-eastern Ontario?

Summary

Practicing as an occupational therapist in the twenty-first century requires an appreciation not only of the illness but also of geographical and ever-evolving social contexts, as well as health care shifts. The recovery paradigm is arguably a good fit with the principles and beliefs of occupational therapy (Rebeiro Gruhl, 2005) and promotes similar social values (Townsend, 1993) for the therapeutic relationship with clients. However, the pragmatics of making this work in therapy remains challenging. These challenges include equitable distribution of resources, system and teams' willingness to include client opinion and experiences in the decision-making process; and, the place of occupation as a valued right of citizenship versus something to do. The issue of social justice, rather than issues of therapy, is likely to be the driving force behind any paradigm shift. This will require occupational therapists to educate, advocate and lobby for the creation of occupational opportunities within their communities.

Meeting the occupational and recovery needs of clients in the community requires an appreciation of the many societal barriers to participation, the paucity of occupational opportunity as well as of the disruptive process of mental illness on occupational engagement and participation in important occupational roles. This disruption serves to alienate the client from many of the benefits derived from direct engagement in occupation (Gould *et al.*, 2005). Furthermore, inadequate funding for mental health systems, stigma regarding mental health consumer capability and competition for limited jobs serve to further marginalise, deprive and alienate mental health consumers from participating in occupation. Subsequently, mental health consumers may be denied the level and depth of participation that is required for their recoveries.

The occupational injustices raised in this chapter may contribute to limited recovery trajectories for many of the study participants and their family members. This dialogue leads to further inquiry about how the system might engage consumers, their families and rural and remote communities into meaningful partnerships and other creative solutions to address these occupational injustices. Occupational injustices may offer one of the best explanations for limited recoveries in north-eastern Ontario and requires further in-depth inquiry to better understand how to position occupational justice as a legitimate variable in the current health care/health promotion dialogue.

This chapter has focused in a specific Canadian context; however, the message for occupational therapists worldwide is that they have a social responsibility to ensure that persons with serious mental illness and other vulnerable people have access to participation in occupation as both therapy and as a right of citizenship. Work is important from many perspectives, and to be denied access to or participation in work is an injustice with grave consequences. Occupational therapists need to create partnerships and collaborative practice so as to manufacture opportunities for participation and for work that offers the support and flexibility required for success.

Questioning your Practice

1. Why is it important for occupational therapists to understand the social values and issues of their community?
2. What are the three things an occupational therapist might do to raise the profile of the need for human occupation in one's community?
3. What are the two ways to increase occupational opportunity in one's community without the benefit of additional human or fiscal resources?

References

Anthony WA (1993) Recovery from mental illness: The guiding vision of the mental health service system in the 1990's. *Psychosocial Rehabilitation Journal, 16(4)*, 11–23.

Anthony WA (2000) A recovery-oriented system: Setting some system level standards. *Psychiatric Rehabilitation Journal, 24(2)*, 159–168.

Cook JV (ed.) (2001) *Qualitative Research in Occupational Therapy*. Albany, NY: Delmar.

Deegan PE (1988) Recovery: The lived experience of rehabilitation. *Psychiatric Rehabilitation Journal, 11*, 11–19.

Erlandsson L-K, Rognvaldsson T, Eklund M (2004) Recognition of similarities: patterns of daily occupations. *Journal of Occupational Science, 11(1)*, 3–13.

Glaser B, Strauss A (1967) *The Discovery of Grounded Theory*. Chicago, IL: Aldine.

Gould A, DeSouza S, Rebeiro Gruhl KL (2005) And then I lost that life: a shared narrative of four young men with schizophrenia. *British Journal of Occupational Therapy, 68(10)*, 1–7.

Hatchard K, Missiuna C (2003) An occupational therapist's journey through bipolar affective disorder. *Occupational Therapy in Mental Health, 19(2)*, 1–17.

Hammell K, Carpenter C (eds) (2003) *Qualitative Research in Evidence-Based Rehabilitation*. Edinburgh: Churchill Livingstone.

Kuhn TS (1970) *The Structure of Scientific Revolution*. (2nd edn). Chicago, IL: The University of Chicago Press.

Legault E, Rebeiro KL (2001) Occupation as means to mental health: A single-case study. *American Journal of Occupational Therapy, 55(1)*, 90–96.

Ministry of Health (2001) *Making It Work: Policy Framework for Employment Supports for People with Serious Mental Illness*. Toronto, ON: Queen's Printer for Ontario.

MacGillivary H, Nelson G (1998) Partnerships in mental health: what it is and how to do it. *Canadian Journal of Rehabilitation, 12(2)*, 71–83.

Nangia P, DiLenardi S, Gasparini J (2005) *Social profile of Greater Sudbury 2004*. Sudbury, ON: Social Planning Council.

Public Health Agency of Canada (1999) *Toward a healthy future: second report on the health of canadians.* http://www.phac-aspc.gc.ca/ph-sp/phdd/report/subin.html. Accessed on 26 Sept 2006.

Rebeiro KL (1998) Occupation as means to mental health. A review of the literature and a call to research. *Canadian Journal of Occupatinal Therapy, 65(1),* 12–19.

Rebeiro KL (1999) The labyrinth of community mental health: in search for meaningful occupation. *Psychiatric Rehabilitation Journal, 23(2),* 143–152.

Rebeiro KL (2000) Client perspectives on occupational therapy practice: are we truly client-centred? *Canadian Journal of Occupational Therapy, 67(1),* 7–14.

Rebeiro KL (2001a) Participant observation as a research strategy. In: JV Cook (ed.) *Qualitative Research in Occupational Therapy: Strategies and Experiences.* Albany, NY: Delmar, pp. 58–74.

Rebeiro KL (2001b) In order to make a difference: A research journey. In: JV Cook (ed.) *Qualitative Research in Occupational Therapy: Strategies and Experiences.* Albany, NY: Delmar, 132–156.

Rebeiro KL (May 2002) MHSIS Institute: Partnerships for Participation in Occupations. Paper presented at American Occupational Therapy Association Annual Conference, USA: Miami, FL.

Rebeiro KL (Nov 2002) Partnerships in Mental Health. Paper presented at Ontario Hospital Association Convention, Canada: Toronto, ON.

Rebeiro KL (May 2004) Recovery Defined from a Northeastern Ontario Perspective. Paper presented at *We All Belong Educational Campaign Meeting,* Canada: Sudbury, ON.

Rebeiro Gruhl KL (2005) Reflections on…the recovery paradigm: should occupational therapists be interested? *Canadian Journal of Occupational Therapy, 72,* 96–102.

Rebeiro Gruhl KL (2006a) Enablers and barriers to recovery: Perspectives from consumers and service providers in Northeastern Ontario. Unpublished manuscript.

Rebeiro Gruhl KL (2006b) Recovery attitudes: Perspectives from consumers, providers and families. Unpublished manuscript.

Rebeiro KL, Allen J (1998) Voluntarism as occupation. *Canadian Journal of Occupational Therapy, 65(5),* 279–85.

Rebeiro KL, Cook JV (1999) Opportunity, not prescription: An exploratory study of the experience of occupational engagement. *Canadian Journal of Occupational Therapy, 66(4),* 176–187.

Rebeiro KL, Day DG, Semeniuk B, O'Brien MC, Wilson B (2001) NISA/Northern Initiative for Social Action: An occupation-based mental health initiative. *American Journal of Occupational Therapy, 55(5),* 493–500.

Statistics Canada (2001) *2001 Census of Population.* Cat No. 97F0024XIE200101B. http://statscan.ca/english. Accessed on 15 Sept 2006.

Strong S, Rebeiro KL (2003) Creation supportive work environments for people with mental illness, (pp. 137–154). In L. Letts, P. Rigby & D. Stewart (Eds) *Using Environments to Enable Occupatinal Performance.* Thorotare NJ: SLAC INC.

Townsend E (1993) Muriel Driver Lecture: Occupational therapy's social vision. *Canadian Journal of Occupational Therapy, 60(4),* 174–84.

Townsend E (1998) *Good Intentions Overruled: A Critique of Empowerment in the Routine Organization of Mental Health Services.* Toronto, ON: University of Toronto Press.

Townsend E (2003) Reflections on Power and justice in enabling occupation. *Canadian Journal of Occupational Therapy, 70(2),* 74–87.

Townsend E, Wilcock AA (2004) Occupational justice and client-centred practice: a dialogue in progress. *Canadian Journal of Occupational Therapy, 71(2),* 75–87.

Wasylenki DA, Goering PN, Lancee WJ, Ballantyne R, Farkas M (1985) Impact of a case management program on psychiatric aftercare. *The Journal of Nervous Mental Disease, 173(5)*, 303–308.

Whiteford G (2000) Occupational deprivation: global challenge in the new millennium. *British Journal of Occupational Therapy, 63(5)*, 200–204.

Wilcock A (1993) A theory of the human need for occupation. *Journal of Occupational Science, 1(1)*, 17–24.

Wright C, Rebeiro KL (2003) Exploration of a single case in a consumer-governed mental health organization. *OT in Mental Health, 19(2)*, 19–32.

9 The art of occupation

Jacqueline Ede

Personal narrative

Living and working in East London, in the UK, it is hard for me to ignore the influence of Walthamstow's William Morris, the nineteenth-century social pioneer and founder of the Arts and Crafts Movement. Morris has easily outlived the mark made by Walthamstow's other famous residents – the 1990s boy band East 17. Importantly, Morris' principles still inspire occupational therapy collaborations with the arts today.

Morris highlights a yearning for freedom that I feel is one of three great motivators alongside empathy and creativity. These notions are all emotive, distinctly human and sadly not always extended towards those people with, or recovering from, mental health difficulties. This can be a source of frustration and a breeding ground for occupational alienation, injustice and deprivation. Our liberty is realised in the ideal of social inclusion: equity, allowance and recognition for all. William Morris was an enthusiastic advocate for fair treatment, better living conditions and the acknowledgment of craftsmanship. He promoted both individualism and collective advantages against soul-less mass production of furnishings, preferring imaginative design. Given his views, it is ironic that his designs have been widely reproduced since his death, although that may reflect their enduring attraction rather than his political opinions.

I consider that empathy is the keenest of driving forces. We all have our mental health alongside our physical and spiritual well-being. However, one in four people will have a mental health problem during their lifetime and most of us will experience, at the very least, the effects of stress, bereavement and anxiety. Fascinated by my own ever-changing emotional state, my work has evolved to a passionate moral support for those much ridiculed and marginalised by society. This has been influenced by working in mental health, over the past 10 years, in psychiatric accident and emergency; acute, low secure and long-stay inpatient units, day hospital and community services.

My third motivator is a strong belief in universal creativity. People are not only occupational beings but also creative beings. Everyday human traits such as problem solving, resourcefulness, invention and flexibility are just as creative as painting, composing music or writing poems. But as occupational therapists how can we truly harness creativity?

Having the opportunity to explore new ground in a practice development occupational therapy post, much of my current work with the arts was founded by the desire to uncover a vehicle for service users to move away from institutions, and their often accompanied staid thinking, to experience greater acceptance in mainstream life. Art has proved a valuable means for this. The success of this approach resulted in the change of my post to focus on leading occupational therapy for the arts and rehabilitation.

Innovation never ceases to amaze the world, but individuals' endeavours can be hidden from view by a lack of access to the elite arts world. For individuals with mental health problems, occupational disruption is caused by clinical symptoms, financial hardship, poor confidence, and resistance resulting from years of invaded privacy and depersonalisation. Yet, mental illness is often linked to the genius of artistic expression as illustrated by the composer Ludwig Van Beethoven, post-impressionist painter Vincent Van Gogh, writer Virginia Woolf and more recently actor Spike Milligan. As Edvard Munch the creator of the painting, *The Scream*, said, '*Without fear and illness, I could never have accomplished all I have*' (Thinkexist, 2007). Reflecting on the ways we may unwittingly curtail ambition brings about greater understanding of how we can broaden existing opportunities and create new openings for people with mental health problems.

After years of running many different creative sessions, using a variety of media including photography, music, writing, craftwork, art and drama, I wondered why the process sometimes seemed demeaning or even patronising for the participants. So, I looked beyond standard review processes, such as participant questionnaires and discussions because of their limited perspectives. They appeared only to ask if people were satisfied with the sessions they had participated in and this generated new ideas for activities, which I would then incorporate into revised sessions. I began to believe that this was tokenistic to client-centred practice, because such a task-orientated approach sets boundaries and limits the realm of possibilities for individuals. Most disturbingly, I recognised I could be perpetuating occupational alienation.

Occupational alienation is addressed more fully in Chapter 7, but it contains elements of isolation, frustration and estrangement leading to a feeling that engagement in occupation does not meet the individual's needs (Wilcock, 1998a). This internal response to activity as an unrewarding experience led me to ask why people went to creative groups. Through detailed discussions, clients identified a range of reasons as to why they attended, including to:

■ relieve boredom;
■ find respite;
■ demonstrate a willingness to get better;
■ show progress;
■ accelerate the chance of discharge;
■ change their mood;
■ be with like-minded people;
■ find a means of expression.

Traditional occupational therapy creative groups have their value and can lend the means to improve health, rediscover latent talent, continue an existing hobby or find a new one; yet occupational alienation can be present. Considering the complexity of initiative, personal drive and decision making, each of the afore-mentioned aims, singly or in combination, potentially holds positive and/or negative traits. Being attentive to participants' motives for engaging in groups is fundamental. If someone is finding involvement in activities anywhere on a scale between uninteresting and soul destroying, this should be investigated to establish the cause, or else there will be the risk of occupational alienation.

To move from running traditional creative groups in the hospital setting, I sought to recognise and showcase the artistic abilities of mental health service users, carers and staff. Hoping to break down some of the barriers that can exist between people, I established a Visual Arts Project in 2003, which is open to all contributions. This was an adjunct to existing occupational therapy services and open to everyone connected with mental health care in the North East London Mental Health Trust (NELMHT). Since April 2006, the project has developed into a budding organisation called thinkarts and its associated reference group Creative Circles. These ventures will be discussed in more detail later.

Occupational potential

Alison Wicks (2001) in a comment paper used an evocative illustration to describe occupational potential; it is worth repeating here.

> A clay pot sitting in the sun all day will always be a clay pot. It has to go through the heat of the furnace to become porcelain (Mildred Witte Stouven, cited in Schaef, 1990, March 30). Actually there is nothing wrong with being a clay pot. It is just all of us have the possibility of becoming porcelain. (Schaef, 1990, cited in Wicks, 2001, p. 32)

Creative activities in occupational therapy

The therapeutic use of the arts can be traced back to classical times, for example, Egyptian writings from as long ago as 2000 BC tell of temples where 'melacholics congregated in large numbers to seek relief... where recreations were instituted' (Turner et al., 1992, p.12).

In the UK the Arts and Crafts Movement instituted by William Morris and others was part of a wider social reform movement, which, according to Wilcock (2001), included Thomas Carlyle, Robert Owen and Octavia Hill. They were all important in the inception of occupational therapy through their influence on Elizabeth Casson, who was instrumental in the development of occupational therapy including establishing the first school of occupational therapy in the UK (Wilcock, 2002). Holder (2001) suggests the tradition association between activity in occupational therapy and crafts derives from these early influences.

Drake (1999, p. 7) credits Tracy in 1910 as the first person to 'designate specific crafts for specific needs'. Also at the turn of the twentieth century, Massachusetts-based doctor Herbert James Hall extolled the virtues of occupation for health by '...combining aims from medicine, psychiatry, the arts, and social work... where patients became "artisans", ... engaging patients in arts and crafts activities' (Quiroga, 1995, p. 93 & 94).

Despite the centrality of occupation as treatment, the profession's historical links to the arts appeared go astray from the 1950s, when there was an identity crisis in the profession as it moved to a more scientific focus to gain more recognition from medicine (Perrin, 2001). In the 1980s, it was acknowledged that creative activities were less valued in treatment programmes (Jungersen, 1981; Swee Hong & Yates, 1995), perhaps suggesting that Western culture favoured cognitive and verbal activities over manual skills. However, the move away from the arts was not to last. Returning to its roots, the profession re-engaged with creative occupations (Perrin, 2001). Other literature, around this time, noted the use of creative occupations in mental health (Craik *et al.*, 1998; Lloyd & Papas, 1999; Griffiths, 2000). The range of creative media used in occupational therapy noted in the literature currently includes digital photography (Fitzgerald, 1999), pottery (Overton Croad, 2002), poetry (Pollard & Steele, 2002) and creative writing (Wood, 2003).

Thus, the profession came full circle with the emergence of occupational science and its emphasis on occupation as central to humans. National occupational therapy associations have moved to define and consolidate their identities based on occupation. Pierce (2003) noted that both the Canadian and the American Association had placed occupation at their philosophical core. The World Federation of Occupational Therapists (WFOT) (2006) definition of occupational therapy emphasises the promotion of health and well-being through occupation, and the WFOT (2002) revision of the curriculum for occupational therapy education placed occupation at the core of professional education.

Although, there is a relative wealth of literature on creative activities and related subjects in occupational therapy, the evidence base of its effectiveness is limited especially, as Lloyd and Papas (1999) highlight, around outcome measurement. Research into the use and efficacy of creative activities was identified in the priority list for occupational therapy in mental health by Fowler Davies and Bannigan (2000) and later by Fowler Davies and Hyde (2002). Although, it did not rate as highly as other issues, it was included.

The art and science of occupation

Through an array of key occupations, people have searched, solved and survived in ever-changing environments, having adapted over time to evolve sophisticated tools for living. There is a fascination with the human capacity to act on their environment, being driven to investigate and create beyond the necessity of survival, for example, earlier cave paintings depicted life at that time but do not appear to have a survival purpose. According to Clapham (1986) the basic needs of the early hunter gatherers were for shelter, warm clothing and tools to get food and water. The occupation of making was vital to providing a home, however temporary, when caves were unavailable, to providing animal skin garments to wear and to construct sharpened materials to catch prey for food. Sadly, for many people in some parts of the world, this focus on occupation for survival persists to the present day.

For other people, making consists of contributing to a larger project such as building bridges, computers, kitchen appliances and fairground attractions as part of their paid employment.

While for another group, their life focus is so remote from occupation in its original meaning that they find ways to include occupation in the everyday life. This is evident, in *Western* society, in the resurgence of lifestyle programmes on television and in magazines promoting the virtues of cooking, gardening and home decoration. However it is achieved, making remains a core occupation.

Through experimenting with occupations people discover who they are. Occupations extend from babies learning to crawl and adolescents testing their independence to adults maintaining their employment and older adults adjusting their occupations to cope with the participation restrictions of later life. This process is achieved over the life span through testing capabilities physically, emotionally and spiritually, by way of trial and error, boundaries and comfort zones are found.

In occupational terms, Nelson (1998) argues that the occupations that people do are both overt and covert. The establishment of an individual's identity and their strengthening sense of self is largely a covert experience, nourished by active occupation, worldly exploration, relations with others, socio-cultural and environmental influences. An individual's sense of self and all that it means is often the springboard for taking opportunities for occupation within the wider environment. These biological attributes in unison with humans' creative capacity have enabled the occupation of making throughout evolution. As occupational therapists, the enjoyment of delving into the arena of people's adaptability to their environment is far too tempting an opportunity to miss, the history of humanity holds many mysteries ripe for unfolding. Engagement in occupation, art specifically, offers participants opportunities for social inclusion, occupational balance and promotion of independence. These will be discussed below, as well as highlighting the place of arts in health.

Social inclusion

The thinkarts project builds on the results from Bryant's (1995) study into long-term, community-based, social contact groups for people with mental health problems. She found that many users preferred these groups to other more formal day care, citing their low-key approach as a reason for this. With its focus away from clinical intervention, thinkarts goes further taking steps to develop community forums called Creative Circles, intended to foster social inclusion. The UK Government's weighty agenda for social inclusion has meant that there is an expectation that those working in the pubic sector will take up the challenge and work towards social inclusion.

Occupational balance

The concept of health as more than the absence of illness is now well established and links to the heart of occupational therapy through occupation's intrinsic connection to well-being since 'man, through the use of his hands as they are energised by mind and will, can influence the state of his own health' (Reilly, 1962, p. 2). It is with this belief that thinkarts endeavours to provide opportunities for users of mental health services, their carers and staff in the NELMHT to promote occupational balance, which leads to well-being (Wilcock, 1998b). A healthy occupational balance should not just include activities of daily living but the unusual and infrequent events that are part of the fabric of life. The thinkarts project aims to give people a choice to participate in its creative ventures to positively affect occupational satisfaction and improve quality of life, which is in keeping with Wilcock's (1998b) view that occupational therapists need to develop new skills in new arenas to develop occupational potential.

Promoting independence

Alongside acknowledging people as occupational beings and utilising occupation to improve quality of life, the concepts of independence, occupational satisfaction, community and social inclusion have been the dominating ideals behind thinkarts. In an American position paper, Hinojosa (2002, p. 7) states that an 'individual's independence should not be based on pre-established criteria, perception of outside observers, or how independence is accomplished'. Promoting independence is a mainstay of thinkarts. Autonomy has been achieved by being person-centred and supportive yet not taking on a clinical or teacher role.

Mocellin (1995) suggested that occupational therapists should exchange occupation for teaching skills as their focus for intervention; Crabtree (1998) countered this view, stating that such an approach has no roots in occupational therapy, as it neglects context and would limit the profession enormously. Furthermore, Crabtree (1998, p. 505) acknowledges that teaching competence-building interventions is important but that it is not as important as 'qualities and characteristics that go beyond skills and competence'. The thinkarts project endeavours to emphasise the characteristics that Crabtree promotes – a state of engagement, a sense of actuality, a sense of authorship and a sense of identity (Crabtree, 1998). Everyone is welcome to contribute to thinkarts, no matter their aptitude and there is no predetermined motive to build skills. Contributors have had to take complete responsibility for engaging, and are buoyed up, if need be, by conversations about their involvement. Furthermore, remaining separate from any hospital service has meant not being associated with any clinical team's identity. Community orientated working and moving away from institutions into the public domain adds to the mainstream characteristic for thinkarts and further develops the arts in health movement.

The arts in health

The Health Education Authority (1999) published a review of good practice in community-based arts projects and interventions which impact on health and well-being. They identified over 200 projects in the UK linked to social or health related issues through intervention in the arts. The thinkarts project follows in this tradition. The Arts Council for England (2002) is involved in ensuring the arts are represented in heath care through a wide range of activities. In addition, there are many other separate arts projects of all different shapes and forms over the country in mental health. These include the START project in Manchester, which employs full-time artists in the occupational therapy-led adult day services, the Bethlem Gallery at the Maudsley Hospital for mental health service users work (Risby & Maddox, 1998), the national Art Works in Mental Health, a partnership of organisations involved in mental health who showcase the creative talents of those with mental health needs, LIME, who work all over health settings in the UK to make the arts a fundamental part of the healing process, and the Arts in Hospital project at Dorset Country Hospital, who borrow contemporary art works to display in public areas. It is against this landscape that thinkarts will be discussed.

Establishing arts projects

The next section of this chapter describes the development of a series of Visual Arts Projects each building on the success of the previous one and each moving further from the confines of hospital services and into the public arena. The impetus for these is based on the themes of occupational science and the practice of occupational therapy, and they will be illustrated in relation to the main themes of the projects.

Financed by the NELMHT charitable fund, a Visual Arts Exhibition was held in 2003 during NHS Week. It involved much partnership working using a new, but as yet unused, ward at Goodmayes Hospital. Practical support was received from a variety of sources and included users of Vocational Rehabilitation and Community Mental Health Teams who helped to set up the exhibition, exercising carpentry, Front of House and interior design skills. Contributors were prepared by being given a detailed fact sheet covering the process, sales options, their rights and the practice development occupational therapist's responsibilities. On display were a variety of works including a rolling poetry display projected on the wall called Poetry in Motion, sculpture, cartoons, textiles, paintings, photographs and drawings by NELMHT service users, carers and staff of all age groups. Many exhibitors sold items of their work, accepted commissions or were invited to teach their expertise to others. The NELMHT produced their 2003–2004 annual report in the form of a calendar illustrated with a selection of works from the exhibition, for which the artists collected a national award.

The exhibition attracted an attendance of over 200 people, and their responses to the event were recorded in the visitor's book. As occupational therapy aims to improve a person's ability to function, increase health, well-being and quality of life through the purposeful use of activities, the entirely positive anecdotes such as 'excellent – really enjoyed it, 'I got so much from this', 'inspired me to re-start my art' and 'more please' indicated its therapeutic value. But it was still too contained within the mental health community. So, the following year, a second Visual Arts Exhibition was held in a more public space, a local theatre attracting more volunteers, contributors and a wider audience.

Creative circles

Following the second exhibition, participants felt there needed to be a way to bring people together to share ideas, plan and organise visual arts events – the first thought was to establish a NELMHT Arts Council. However, the name seemed too formal and better suited to a chaired committee. Therefore, many versions later, the name of Creative Circle was agreed upon to promote the notion of equality and shared leadership. The aim of the Creative Circles is to serve as a reference group for all arts activities providing regular feedback and adding a greater element of accountability. In keeping with the aim of inclusively, a logo for this group has been created by a service user and acts as the identification mark on all promotional and advertising flyers and materials. Membership has been drawn from service users, staff and carers with interests and talents in creative pursuits as varied as music, stand-up comedy, poetry reading, amateur dramatics, graphic design, textiles, art and crafts. Meetings are held at community venues such as theatres, town halls and galleries.

To progress from this stage, it was necessary to contend with the concept of outsider art. The term was noted by Roger Cardinal and is applied to the output of people who have no supposed artistic background. As outsider artists have had no conditioning, they show purity of expression. However, the term can be misused or misunderstood, especially by those who use mental health services, who may consider it to be demeaning. As one in four people experience a mental health problem, the term applies to a quarter of all trained or untrained artists, whether they are involved in conventional settings or not. Where would this leave a twenty-first-century dwelling Van Gogh? To remove the straitjackets and labels that exist in both the arts and health, perhaps other terms such as 'Free Art' or 'Open Art' would be more appropriate terminology to honour those taking their own work beyond traditional routes and enable greater occupational satisfaction (Ede, as cited in O'Reilly *et al.*, 2006).

To move further into the mainstream, the next step was to ascertain whether any London-based arts facilities would like to team up with the NELMHT. The Serpentine Gallery in Kensington Gardens, a famous location in central London, responded positively, and a meeting with their educational programmers resulted in an enthusiastic agreement to work together. Initially project workshops were hosted at the Serpentine Gallery for service users and staff to join with artists to visit their exhibitions regularly, responding to use of the artistic media and to explore ideas related to the display. These also provided forums to discuss future partnership working.

Hearing voices, seeing things

The partnership with the Serpentine Gallery grew from recognising the appetite for creativity in the mental health service user community and the frustrating inability to access the mainstream art world. Over a 3-year period a programme called Hearing Voices, Seeing Things developed with funding from The Big Lottery Fund, Rayne Foundation and Bloomberg, through a series of seven projects involving 150 people.

Adolescents designed images on plates donated by the world famous manufacturers Wedgewood for the grand fete event the Crockery Smash Up with ceramist Karen Densham. Young carers explored their home ground with new eyes in a photographic project called Urban Jungle with Andy Lawson. Hearing Voices Group members informed and contributed to the psychosis experience instillations of Silent Interruptions with Victor Mount. People with dementia created a new alphabet and lyrical works for Reminder with Bob and Roberta Smith. Adults of working age made a radio show in Ha Ha Bonk Telling Stories through Sound Effects with Mel Brimfield and Sally O'Reilly, and they created a theatre-based tableaux with Mandy Lee Jandrell and enjoyed plenty of humour through 'What's So Funny?' with Jessica Voorsanger.

The projects culminated with a month-long Hearing Voices, Seeing Things exhibition at the Serpentine Gallery in autumn 2006. A collection of three posters were created with the London Transport's art organisation, Platform for Art, to advertise the event and were shown across the London Underground tube network. A book detailing and illustrating each project, with additional contributions from poet and service user John Hegley and psychoanalyst Darian Leader was launched at the exhibition. The exhibition was an opportunity not only for those not directly involved in the projects to celebrate their innovative contribution to the art world, but also, for the viewers to question and challenge their preconceptions about mental health. The exhibition opening night was extremely well attended and generated a great deal of excitement and positive reviews. This approach of working closely with the arts has continued to be developed.

The thinkarts project and vocational opportunities

As a result of these initiatives and increased interest, it was necessary to create an umbrella organisation to further this work and encourage arts-related events, projects, voluntary and freelancing opportunities for people who have experienced mental ill health. Recognising the talent and expertise of mental health service users, alongside the barriers often experienced by individuals when accessing the world of art and business, thinkarts was founded in April 2006. Thinkarts endeavours to decrease exclusion by developing healthy and mutually beneficial partnerships with organisations in the wider community. Currently affiliated to the NELMHT, the organisation is working towards becoming an independent social enterprise.

Prior to, and throughout, thinkarts' lifetime, service users have sought out opportunities to be involved in arts work, providing the inspiration, energy and ideas for projects, shaping the way forward to where we are today. Through thinkarts, individuals are forming a collective able to respond to requests from the community, spanning user groups to commercial businesses, education facilities to charities, for artworks and activities, for example, producing logos and advertising, or using skills to run sessions for local community groups.

The thinkarts project can be a learning ground providing work experience opportunities for those who are seeking employment or fulfilling their vocational needs outside paid work. It caters to all people irrespective of their work status or current activities. This is particularly important as the National Institute for Mental Health in England (NIMHE) (2003) suggests that over half a million people with mental health problems are not seeking work or are considered to be permanently sick. As the UK Government's ambition is to achieve social inclusion, addressing the issue of unemployment is imperative. In the UK, occupational therapists appear to have neglected the vocational aspect of the profession in recent years and have focused on other aspects of rehabilitation. Further, exploration of this is found in Chapter 10.

With funding from Capital Volunteering, London's pilot organisation to increase volunteering opportunities in mental health, thinkarts' members of all ages and backgrounds have benefited from being involved as volunteers or participants in a wide variety of activities. These have included organising and invigilating Paint the Town Red, a World Mental Health Art Exhibition, teaching pastel and batik workshops, responding to graphic design commissions,; enjoying sessions with poets and craft specialists, assembling and rotating the *Poems in the Waiting Room* collection across clinic reception areas, building the thinkarts Web site and producing regular newsletters. It is hoped that the 'thinkarts newsletter' will become a glossy magazine that will continue to be free to service users and voluntary organisation on subscription, but will be sold externally through art galleries and bookshops.

Members have the opportunity to progress from volunteering to being paid either as freelancers or via permitted earnings, therefore protecting their benefit status. Some of the specific paid roles currently filled are events photographers, report writers, interviewers, publication layout specialists, carpenters and Web site developers. As illustrated, thinkarts is in a position to provide a wealth of opportunities for those who gain enjoyment and improved occupational well-being from engaging in creative pursuits.

Case Study 9.1 Pete's narrative

I am a long-term mental health service user and have problems with my moods and depression for which I take mood stabilisers and anti-depressants when needed. I attend a day centre for people with mental health problems for 2 days per week doing pottery and art therapy. The art therapist there put me in touch with thinkarts.

I am very interested in graphics especially computer art; so thinkarts commissioned me to do several pieces of work: firstly, a board game called 'Well-Travelled' created as an accompaniment for NELMHT's annual report, and postcard flyers and ten-way markers for a mile-long walking circuit at Goodmayes Hospital. I have also been involved with thinkarts Web presence and am currently developing an events calendar for the site.

This has been a real lifesaver for me, as I felt that my artwork had no value and was going nowhere. Doing work with and for thinkarts has made me feel a lot better about myself, and my feelings of self-worth have been raised a few notches. I have been to workshops and visits arranged by thinkarts, which have motivated me to leave my flat and get some much-needed personal interaction. It has helped me gain confidence in dealing with people and my surrounding *milieu*.

Case Study 9.2 Caroline's narrative

It is the support of institutions, friends and family that helps keep one focused on the steep hill that people of mental health have to climb – one must soldier on, create a routine and understand that one will go through patches of utter despair, but with motivation and determination, it has to be possible to reach the summit. I have to go through all the basics of life all over again – building self-esteem, confidence and a sense of worth, and with that, the desire to enjoy the creative part of my being slowly comes back.

With the help of thinkarts I have really appreciated and enjoyed being involved in projects, such as Hearing Voices, Seeing Thing,: The Tableaux and What's so Funny? These were so important at the time to give one a direction and make one feel wanted. I then wished to move on from being an actor to a producer; as I used to make a living from sculpting metals and wood, making my own art again is my ultimate aim.

To brush up my skills I went on a local college's welding course and am enjoying going to the thinkarts studio, where I am working on a piece of cherry wood, which gives me pleasure and purpose. Currently I am looking to share a studio with another sculptor.

Extending occupational therapy

It can be considered that in occupational therapy there are two models of professionalism, technical rational and practical artistry, which need not be pitted against one another. Rather, there should be an acceptance of the need for both knowledge and imagination and that these are not divisions of science and arts but are fundamentally linked. The shift in the profession towards evidence-based practice could be seen to favour the technical rational approach and perhaps links to the move away from the creative activities in the past, as they may have been judged to lack scientific rigour. However, the development of occupational science and the recent work such as Reynolds (2002) and Schmid (2004) using qualitative methodology may have shifted the balance back in favour of the relevance of creative activities.

The joint publication by the College of Occupational Therapists and Royal College of Psychiatrists (2002, p. 7) recognises that occupational therapists have the 'capacity to apply activity and meaningful occupation as a therapeutic tool to the benefit of individuals'. But, the location of that activity does not have to be in a hospital or care setting. Increasingly occupational therapists are moving beyond their traditional boundaries to extend their work into a wider arena. Creek (2002) noted that few occupational therapists work with the well population. The thinkarts project, by supporting staff, who are delivering purposeful creative groups, aims to consolidate benefits to health. Although, in health promotion literature, work–life balance has often been ignored, as confirmed by Howell and Pierce (2000), who suggest that, in the West, work is prized more than rest and the restorative value of occupation is not acknowledged. This experimental arena will require greater study to provide an evidence base for it, and thinkarts can be a vehicle to do so.

Working as part of a multi-professional organisation, it is important that others are able to understand the role of occupational therapy. However, Kaur *et al.* (1996) found that other professionals recognised the role of occupational therapy in mental health in relation to activities of daily living, but they were less clear about other aspects including the use of creative activities. This may limit the referral of potential clients to occupational therapy and prevent them from benefiting from engagement in such occupations. Working with the arts can advertise loud and proud how occupational therapists can use both the process and the fruits of creative activities in public fields.

Summary

The link between the arts and occupational therapy has a long history, although at times it has not received as much recognition as it has during other times. The development of occupational science has enabled the profession to focus on occupation and has reinforced its place at the centre of the profession. Recent literature has described a variety of creative arts used in occupational therapy, and research using qualitative methodology has highlighted the benefits that clients attribute to engaging in creative occupations. Through the arts, there are opportunities to extend the professions' influence beyond its traditional boundaries and to bring the benefits of creativity and occupation to a wider range of people. It seems appropriate that creativity has been employed in the development of these innovations, and they provide examples for other areas of the profession.

Questioning your Practice

1. When does the use of the arts move from clinical intervention to art for art's sake?
2. How far should occupational therapy extend into the wider fields such as the arts?
3. Should projects such as thinkarts be optional extras or key provisions for mental health services?

References

Arts Council of England (2002) *Arts in Healthcare*. London: Arts Council.

Bryant W (1995) The social contact group: an example of long-term group work in community mental health care. *British Journal of Occupational Therapy, 58(5)*, 214–218.

FM (1986) *History of the World*. London: Grisewood & Dempsey Limited.

College of Occupational Therapists and Royal College of Psychiatrists (2002) *Mental Health and Occupation in Participation*. London: College of Occupational Therapists & Royal College of Psychiatrists.

Crabtree JL (1998) Occupational therapy: building skills or transforming selves? *British Journal of Occupational Therapy, 61(11)*, 504–508.

Craik C, Chacksfield JD, Richards G (1998) A survey of occupational therapy practitioners in mental health. *British Journal of Occupational Therapy, 61(5)*, 227–34.

Creek J (2002) *Occupational Therapy & Mental Health*. 3rd ed. Edinburgh: Churchill Livingstone.

Drake M (1999) *Crafts in Therapy and Rehabilitation*. (2nd ed.). USA: Slack Incorporated.

Fitzgerald P (1999) Digital photography and occupational therapy. *Occupational Therapy News, 8*, 14.

Fowler Davies S, Bannigan K (2000) Priorities in mental health research: the results of a live research project. *British Journal of Occupational Therapy, 63(3)*, 98–104.

Fowler Davies S, Hyde P (2002) Priorities in mental health research: an update. *British Journal of Occupational Therapy, 65(8)*, 387–389.

Griffiths S (2000) *The Clinical Utility of Creative Activities used as an Occupational Therapy Treatment Medium for People with Mental Health Problems*. Oxford: MSc.

Health Education Authority (1999) *Art for Health*. London: Health Education Authority.

Hinojosa J (2002) Broadening the construct of independence. *American Journal of Occupational Therapy, 56(6)*, 7.

Holder V (2001) The use of creative activities within occupational therapy. *British Journal of Occupational Therapy, 64(2)*, 103–105.

Howell D, Pierce D (2000) Exploring the forgotten restorative dimension of occupation: quilting and quilt use. *Journal of Occupational Science, 7(2)*, 68–72.

Jungersen K (1981) *The Use & Importance of Activity in Occupational Therapy. A Review of the Literature and Practice*. New Zealand: Dip, Central Institute of Technology.

Kaur D, Seager M, Orrell M (1996) Occupation or therapy? The attitudes of mental health professionals. *British Journal of Occupational Therapy, 59(7)*, 319–322.

Lloyd C, Papas V (1999) Art as therapy within occupational therapy in mental health settings: a review of the literature. *British Journal of Occupational Therapy, 62(1)*, 31–35.

Mocellin G (1995) Occupational therapy: a critical overview, part 1. *British Journal of Occupational Therapy, 58(12)*, 502–506.

National Institute for Mental Health in England (2003) *Employment for People with Mental Health Problems*. London: National Institute for Mental Health in England.

Nelson DL (1998) Occupation: form and performance. *American Journal of Occupational Therapy, 42(10)*, 633–641.

O'Reilly S, Coysh L, Ede JA, Leader D (2006) *Hearing Voices, Seeing Things*. London: Serpentine Gallery.

Overton T, Croad R (2002) The Gemini project: OT and 'the arts'. *Occupational Therapy News, 10,* 27.

Perrin T (2001) Don't despise the funny bunny: a reflection from practice. *British Journal of Occupational Therapy, 64(3),* 129–134.

Pierce D (2003) How can the occupation base of occupational therapy be strengthened? *Australian Occupational Therapy Journal,* 50 1-2.

Pollard N, Steele A (2002) From Doncaster to Dumfries Mental health & poetry events. *Occupational Therapy News, 10,* 31.

Quiroga VAM (1995) *Occupational Therapy: The First 30 Years 1900-1930.* Bethesda, USA: America Occupational Therapy Association Inc.

Reilly M (1962) Occupational therapy can be one of the great ideas of 20th century medicine. *American Journal of Occupational Therapy, 16(1),* 1–9.

Reynolds F (2002) Symbolic aspects of coping with chronic illness through textile arts. *The Arts in Psychotherapy, 29(2),* 99–106.

Risby K, Maddox I (1998) The New Bethlem Art Gallery. *Mental Health OT, 3(3),* 13–15.

Schmid T (2004) Meanings of creativity within occupational therapy practice. *Australian Occupational Therapy Journal, 51(2),* 80–88.

Swee Hong C, Yates P (1995) Purposeful activities? What are they? *British Journal of Occupational Therapy, 58(2),* 75–76.

Thinkexist (2007) http://thinkexist.com/quotes/edvard_munch/ Accessed on 1 Feb 2007.

Turner A, Foster M, Johnson SE (1992) *Occupational Therapy for Physical Dysfunction.* England: Churchill Livingstone.

Wicks A (2001) Occupational potential: a topic worthy of exploration. *Journal of Occupational Science, 8(3),* 32–35.

Wilcock A (1998b) *An Occupational Perspective of Health.* New Jersey: Slack Incorporated.

Wilcock A (1998a) Occupation for health. *British Journal of Occupational Therapy, 61(8),* 340–345.

Wilcock A (2001) *Occupation for Health; A Journey from Self Health to Prescription.* London: College of Occupational Therapists.

Wilcock A (2002) *Occupation for Health; A Journey from Prescription to Self Health.* London: College of Occupational Therapists.

Wood J (2003) The writing's on the wall. *Mental Health Occupational Therapy, 8(1),* 32–33.

World Federation of Occupational Therapists (2002) *Revised Minimum Standards for the Education of Occupational Therapists.* Forrestfield, Australia: WFOT.

World Federation of Occupational Therapists (2006) http://www.wfot.org.au/information.asp Accessed on 28 Nov. 2006.

10 Vocational rehabilitation in the UK
How occupational therapy can contribute

Carla van Heerden

Personal narrative

My journey as an occupational therapist started 20 years ago, 2000 miles away from where I am writing today. Many aspects have changed while other aspects have stayed, surprisingly, the same. In writing this chapter, I hope to share some of the experiences I have had throughout my career and highlight some of the issues that have had an impact on the choices I have made along the way. I shall try to reflect on those aspects that stayed the same, throughout many changes in terms of work context, place and policy. I think these are the powerful messages from occupational therapy philosophy that have become embedded within my personal set of values to shape the meaning of occupation in my own life. I shall introduce some of these influences briefly, as I recall the story of my career, before revisiting them later as I try to explain how they contribute to my current practice.

I studied occupational therapy at the University of the Free State, in Bloemfontein, South Africa, between 1984 and 1988. The work of Vona du Toit, a South African occupational therapist who developed the Model of Creative Ability (Du Toit, 1974), was taught on the course at the time. This model, applicable to all conditions within the spectrum of health care, emphasises the relationship between human volition and action and how this relationship can be used by occupational therapists to understand engagement in activity. Comprehensively written, the model offers information on assessment as well as treatment in occupational therapy, emphasising the centrality of activity as the operational medium for the profession. This model has influenced my work to the extent that it is at times difficult to distinguish which aspects of my practice are not related to it.

Moving on from my student days, my first post as an occupational therapist was in a large general hospital that offered a wide spectrum of possibilities in terms of clinical opportunities. Working with clients who had spinal cord injuries provided a valuable experience of following a small group of patients from the acute stage of disability throughout their rehabilitation. This happened because of my move from the spinal cord unit within the hospital to community services at more or less the same time that the patients made the same move. It was through this holistic experience that I recognised my interest in mental health as I was consistently drawn to and intrigued by the social, emotional and psychological issues confronting this group of young, African men whom I came to know so well. As their community occupational therapist, I was involved in working with the group to match their skills with local needs so as to find sustainable vocational opportunities. Within the political and economic climate at the time, jobs had to be created, rather than applied for, as unemployment figures were high, even amongst those without disability. The group and I were successful in securing a contract with the local casino to produce rattan fruit baskets. I have often used this story to illustrate how any activity can be meaningful within the appropriate context, even though occupational therapists are frequently embarrassed about their basket-weaving heritage.

My next post was in a private, acute psychiatric hospital. I enjoyed developing my skills as a mental health occupational therapist and I conducted a research project exploring the role of the occupational therapist during initial assessment. Job retention and liaison with employers were common features of the post, as the average length of stay in the hospital was 2 weeks. To cope with the fast turnover of clients, I developed a group assessment based on the Model of Creative Ability (Du Toit, 1974).

From here I moved to private practice, first in a multi-disciplinary setting, focusing on mental health in an urban community, with a proportion of work being centred on mental health at work, offering stress management courses to local businesses and schools. Next, we moved as a family to a rural community where I worked as a single practitioner offering a wide range of services including consultation work for a non-government organisation. It was during this time that I decided to study sensory integration theory, as many of the referrals to private occupational therapists in South Africa are children and I thought that it would be wise to satisfy the market need. My experience in mental health, however, drew my attention to the relationship between the sensory processing theories that I was learning and the mental health conditions I had come across before. It was not long before this interest developed and I started researching, informally, how this theory impacts on human behaviour at all stages of development.

I have been working in the field of mental health since moving to England with my family in 1998, and I am currently researching the clinical reasoning of occupational therapists who apply sensory integration theory in their work with adults who have insecure attachment styles. My current post is that of consultant occupational therapist for employment and vocational opportunities across two Mental Health Trusts in the north and east of London and London South Bank University.

In the UK, the role of consultant therapist in the National Health Service was introduced in the NHS Plan (Department of Health, 2000a) and amplified in the strategy for allied health professions (Department of Health, 2000b), which set out to acknowledge and support the development of innovative practice and career development structures. According to this document, the core functions of the consultant therapist are to modernise services, deliver clinical expertise, develop education, training and learning opportunities, support evidence-based practice and research and offer strategic and professional leadership.

Applying these core functions in the field of employment and vocational opportunities allows me to work holistically and integrate the experiences I have had in
the past. Before sharing some aspects of my current role, it is, however, necessary
to consider the background against which employment and vocational services for
persons with mental health problems are being developed.

Vocational rehabilitation

Since 2004, several policy documents published in the UK have cited the relationships between unemployment and health. The direction of these political drivers,
are summarised with this quote:

> By 2025, disabled people in Britain should have full opportunities and choices to improve
> their quality of life and will be respected and included as equal members of society. (Prime
> Minister's Strategy Unit, 2005)

This vision statement highlighted the current lack of opportunity, choice, quality
of life and social inclusion of disabled people and stated an intention to rectify the
situation over the next two decades. Employment and vocational opportunities
are the key features of social participation and quality of life (ODPM, 2004), and
in achieving this vision, access to meaningful employment must be addressed.
Figures show that those with mental health problems have the lowest rate of
employment among those classified with some form of disability, and that only
21% of persons with long-term mental health problems are in work (ODPM, 2004).
Five main reasons for this have been identified by the Social Exclusion Report
(ODPM, 2004). These include stigma and discrimination (fewer than 4 in 10
employers would employ someone who declares having a mental health problem); low expectations of health and social care professionals; a lack of clear
responsibility for promoting vocational and social outcomes for persons with
mental health problems; a lack of ongoing support to facilitate work; and barriers
to engage in the community through using transport services, or having access to
community centres or housing in areas where these services are provided.

It is alarming for occupational therapists, who consider meaningful participation in occupation as central to their practice (Creek, 2003), to hear that the low
expectations of health professionals have been identified as one of the main contributors to the social exclusion of people with mental health problems. The College of Occupational Therapists has, however, taken action to position the
profession at the core of implementing changes on a national level, through becoming official partners to the National Social Inclusion Programme (ODPM, 2004).
This programme was introduced to drive and coordinate the efforts of all mental
health services to actively promote social inclusion.

In north-east London, striving towards more socially inclusive outcomes for
people with mental health problems has become a high priority for the two service
providers; the North East London Mental Health Trust (NELMHT) and the East

London and City Mental Health Trust (ELCMHT). Together these providers offer mental health services to a population close to 1.5 million people. The role of the consultant occupational therapist for employment and vocational opportunities is to ensure that addressing the employment and vocational needs of service users becomes embedded into all aspects of the mental health services provided. Occupational therapy services act as champions for the work.

The role of occupational therapy in the strategy for employment and vocational services in north-east London

The Routes 2 Employment project (R2E) led the way in terms of employment and vocational service provision in NELMHT and ELCMHT. This project has two main aims to address employer practices as well as health care practices. Ultimately, the project hopes to provide more opportunities for people with mental health problems to be included, through employment, as equal members of society.

In terms of employer practices, a toolkit, titled 'Positive about mental health' (Colson & Howells, 2005) was produced, which outlines standards of good practice in terms of employing people with mental health problems. Using this toolkit across the two trusts has resulted in better practices regarding their recruitment and retention policies, including a more proactive stance in creating employment opportunities for service users within the service itself.

The project further outlined a strategy to ensure that employment and vocational services are developed within the existing service structures, using occupational therapy as the lead profession. An employment and vocational opportunity (EVO) lead occupational therapist was identified in each of the (seven) London boroughs covered by NELMHT and ELCMHT, creating a virtual team in each of the two trusts. The consultant occupational therapist meets regularly with each team to discuss service development, clinical issues and cascade information to them. They, in turn, take this to their specific areas of work, and the knowledge they have gained is again shared and distributed. This structure tasks occupational therapists with playing an active role in service development, with an expectation that they should be knowledgeable about the local employment market and other employment service providers in the area. They also need to become involved in, or initiate, projects that could create opportunities for those using mental health services. In addition, they need to have the clinical confidence to provide employment and vocational services, and understand what this means within the context of the service setting where they are working.

Occupational therapists as providers of employment and vocational services

According to current evidence, better employment outcomes are achieved for those with severe mental health problems when they are supported in employment

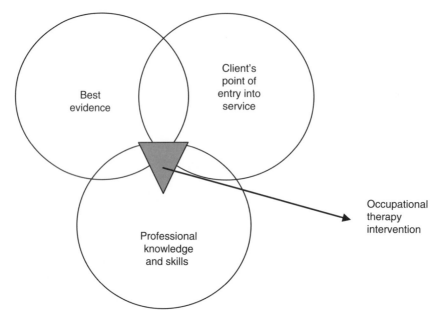

Figure 10.1   Factors influencing occupational therapists' decision-making in vocational rehabilitation.

situations than when they receive pre-vocational training (Crowther *et. al.*, 2001). The Individual Placement and Support Approach (Bond, 2004), which involves a quick assessment of vocational skills and aspirations, followed by active efforts to find placements in suitable employment settings and then providing ongoing support, is advocated as the way forward for the provision of vocational services in the UK (National Social Inclusion Programme, 2006).

Several factors impact on occupational therapists' decision making when they become involved in delivering employment and vocational services. They need to balance the vocational needs of their individual clients at the point of entry into the mental health service with the current evidence and their professional skills as occupational therapists (Figure 10.1).

The individual placement and support approach has been instrumental in making vocational rehabilitation services more relevant to the social inclusion agenda, as it involves active efforts to find suitable placement opportunities in 'real life' situations (National Social Inclusion Programme, 2006). To occupational therapists, this approach should not constitute newly acquired knowledge. As early as 1968, Du Toit, a South African occupational therapist and author of the Model of Creative Ability, specified three basic principles of occupational therapy as being (1) that the individual is treated as a totality; (2) that intervention is by means of the patient's active participation in selected and graded purposeful activity; and (3) that the restoration of the residual work capacity of the individual, or its nearest equivalent, is identified as the fundamental aim of intervention. Nearly 40 years later, occupational therapists have accumulated experiences and knowledge in this field, which they could contribute to the current situation. Descriptions of the individual placement and support approach involve details on service structures, such as integrating vocational programmes into the work of the clinical team or health service or to offer time-unlimited support tailored to individual need (Bond, 2004). What is not described is the content of the support offered, or how to help someone identify vocational goals if this is something they have not considered before. It is in these areas that occupational therapists can offer valuable knowledge. Some of this knowledge is shared in the context of the employment and vocational services offered by occupational therapists in north-east London. They are faced with three key questions when considering their role:

- How are employment/vocational opportunities defined?
- How are vocational issues addressed at different points of entry into the mental health service; for example, how do we approach employment and vocational opportunities on an acute ward, as opposed to in a community mental health team?
- How can the support offered be graded to encourage independence and recovery?

These questions will now be considered in turn.

Defining employment/vocational opportunities

The need to define employment and vocational opportunities stems from the need to define the outcomes of occupational therapy in this field. It would be difficult to determine the effectiveness of the service without first agreeing on what is to be achieved. From a political perspective, there is a strong drive to improve the chances of people with mental health problems gaining access to paid employment. Although this is challenging, individuals may have different vocational aspirations and there is more than one route towards achieving these.

Taylor (2003) takes Glucksmann's TSOL (1995) and develops it to provide a framework for understanding work (see Figure 10.2). This begins with the assumption that work or productivity is an activity that involves the production of goods for use by others, provides a service to others or can be performed by someone other than the one benefiting from it (Taylor, 2003). It then conceptualises work within its social context, through identifying different sectors within society, where these activities could take place. Private, public, formal and informal aspects of work are acknowledged and situated on a continuum, which indicate that they are not distinctly separable from one another. Within each of these sectors, one can further be doing either paid or unpaid work.

Plotting the different sectors creates a visual representation of the broad spectrum of sectors where work can take place. When an individual's work activities are mapped within this framework, the interconnections between the different sectors become more evident (Taylor, 2003). In the context of mental health practice, the classification system could help service users to identify in which sector they are currently working and how they could move to another sector if they wished. It becomes possible to identify how skills can be transferred and to recognise how their current productive activity has meaning within a social context.

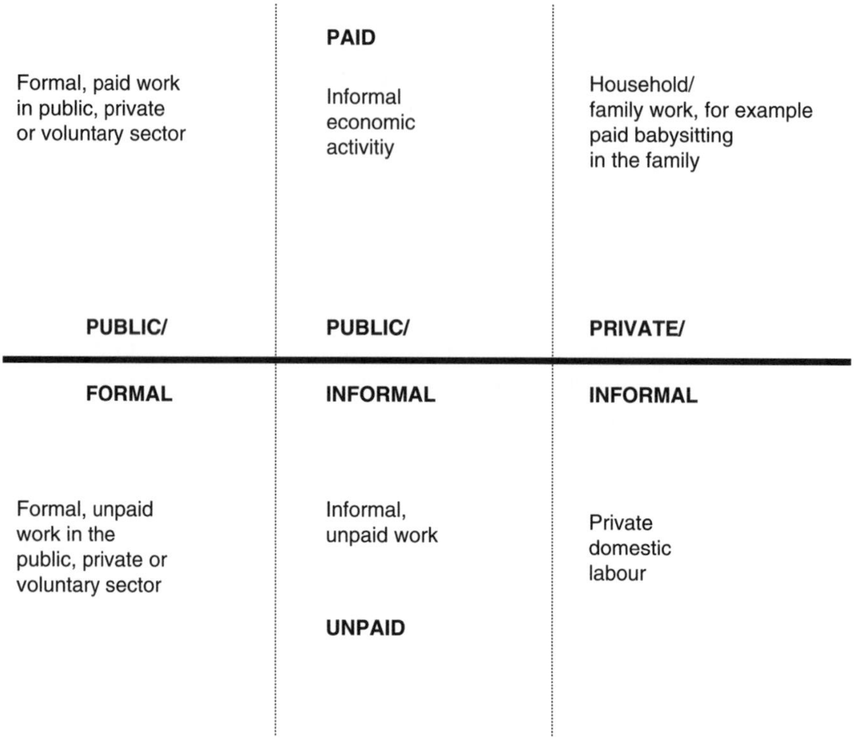

	PAID	
Formal, paid work in public, private or voluntary sector	Informal economic activitiy	Household/ family work, for example paid babysitting in the family
PUBLIC/	**PUBLIC/**	**PRIVATE/**
FORMAL	**INFORMAL**	**INFORMAL**
Formal, unpaid work in the public, private or voluntary sector	Informal, unpaid work	Private domestic labour
	UNPAID	

Figure 10.2   The organisation of labour in society. With permission from Taylor (2003).

Recording individual service users' movement between and across different sectors would allow the service to reflect a true picture of the vocational needs and aspirations of its clients. This data could be helpful when trying to understand the journey that clients travel in achieving their employment and vocational goals. It also becomes possible to record the interim vocational targets achieved, should a client for example desire to work in the paid, public and formal sector, but during the first quarter of the year managed to move from informal, unpaid work to paid informal economic activity.

Addressing vocational issues at different points of entry into the service

The ideal to embed vocational services into mainstream service provision can only be realised if everyone who enters the service has an equal opportunity to be asked about their vocational goals and aspirations. As the Social Exclusion Unit identified (ODMP, 2004), there is a temptation to revert to low expectations when someone is acutely unwell as practitioners may find it hard to know what their roles are at different stages of the recovery process.

The recovery process has been described as a dynamic journey, which could be understood in terms of four stages (Mahler *et al.*, 2001). Two concepts are used to name and demarcate the stages. These are the individual's level of dependence on services or others and the individual's awareness of the relationship between mental health status and degree of control in the process of recovery. A person's status in terms of these two aspects, the role clinicians in mental health services could play and roles for community support systems are outlined for each of four stages as dependent/unaware; dependent/aware; independent/aware and interdependent/aware. Although individuals would not necessarily follow from one stage to another stage sequentially in a neatly organised or developmental sequence, the stages help to identify a person's recovery status at any point of entry into the mental health service.

Clinicians have found an understanding of different stages of recovery helpful in raising their positive expectations of clients, especially during the early stages of recovery. Using the guidelines provides structure to their thinking and it becomes possible to facilitate small steps towards increased awareness and greater independence from the onset of their contact with mental health services. On one admission ward, staff developed a screening questionnaire to identify which clients wanted to receive advice and support in terms of employment or vocation. The staff was surprised to find that eight out of the nine clients on the ward, at the time, indicated that they would be interested in talking to someone about employment, in spite of the staff initially considering that their stage of illness was too acute to have these discussions.

Grading support to promote recovery

As mentioned earlier, the role of the occupational therapist in the field of employment and vocational opportunities remains that of a therapist, rather than an employment specialist. Although the desired outcomes, to achieve vocational goals, are the same, occupational therapists still integrate theoretical approaches, through the process of clinical reasoning, into the actions they take when negotiating with their clients on how to progress towards achieving their goals. Whilst the impact of illness on the client is impairing his or her ability to make fully independent decisions, the occupational therapist will adjust the demands made on the person and make decisions that should eventually develop increased autonomy for the client (Creek, 2003).

The Model of Creative Ability

To meet the challenges of knowing when to steer clients in a certain direction and when to let go so that they can have more autonomy, the Model of Creative Ability (Du Toit, 1972), mentioned in the introduction, offers useful guidelines. Although the model is too comprehensive to fully share within the context of this chapter, some of its tenets that apply in this context are summarised in this section.

Philosophically, the Model of Creative Ability is based on phenomenological and existential principles and is developmentally organised (De Witt, 2005).

The term 'creative ability' refers to the ability to perform, without anxiety, those occupational behaviours one freely chooses to engage in (Du Toit, 1991). This definition implies that the theory is concerned with the development of human volition as the choice, will or drive to engage in activity. A core concept is that each individual has a certain capacity to act creatively, in all spheres of life. This capacity represents the person's potential for development or recovery. At any point in time, this capacity is at a certain stage of being fulfilled or not.

Movement from current level of creative ability towards creative capacity through exerting creative effort

The theory holds that people move through different levels of creative ability, until creative capacity is reached (Figure 10. 3). These levels are identified in a developmental sequence, based on how people are propelled towards the engagement in certain actions through the normal process of human development. In the initial stages described by Du Toit's (1974) model, the relationship between intellectual and motor development is closely associated with that of volition, with differences becoming more evident at the later stages. Du Toit (1974) emphasises the relationship between volition and action, with action being the visible component, or culmination, of volition. Trauma, illness or disease can impede upon this development or the ability to function as close to one's creative capacity as considered ideal.

Table 10.1 lists the levels of motivation, and their corresponding levels of action as described in the model.

The role of the therapist in applying this theory is to determine the client's current level of creative ability, through careful observation and interpretation of the

Table 10.1 Levels of action and corresponding levels of motivation, as described in the Model of Creative Ability

Level of action	Level of motivation
Pre-destructive	Tone
Destructive Incidentally constructive	Self-differentiation
Explorative	Self-presentation
Experimental	Passive participation
Imitative	Imitative participation
Original	Active participation
Competitive	Competitive participation
Situation-centred	Contribution
Society-centred	Competitive contribution

Source: From Du Toit (1974).

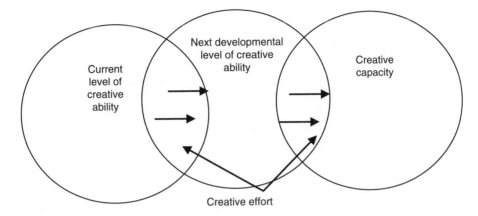

Figure 10.3   Transition from a level of creative ability to creative capacity.

actions performed by the client. It is then necessary to estimate the client's creative capacity, and this is achieved through talking to the client about life goals and ambitions, as well as gathering information about past achievements and preferred activities before the onset of illness. Following this, the therapist would begin to engage the client in activities, chosen to correspond with the current level of creative ability. This important principle changes the perspective of the therapist from using a personal set of values to select suitable treatment media, to a guided approach, following the client's level of motivation. In practice, applying this principle means that language such as 'the client is not motivated to attend therapy sessions', does not exist; rather, the task of the therapist is to discover what the client is motivated to do, and present opportunities to engage in such activities. At the point of engagement, a new challenge emerges for the therapist. If there is to be movement towards the direction of creative capacity, it will be necessary that the client exert creative effort, indicated in Figure10. 3, on the outer boundaries of the circle representing creative ability. This implies that the therapist needs to continually grade and adapt the activity requirements, presenting an ongoing challenge to the client, which is not far enough away from his or her own level of motivation to result in disengagement but not so easy that the demands of the activity are met effortlessly. Throughout this process, the therapist needs to be continually aware of the needs of the client, as well as his or her role in the therapy situation. The therapeutic relationship is structured as one where the therapist sometimes leads (termed the therapist-directed phase) and sometimes follows (the patient-directed phase) the process to maintain the therapeutic milieu and set the appropriate level of challenge. The rules and boundaries are clear but the rules may include role reversal and an ability, on the part of the therapist, to have difficult, honest conversations about personal experiences in the relationship and how the client's engagement is perceived. The client is always enlisted in the process of linking past, present and future to make sense of the engagement process and its relevance to the their overall goal.

Using this model therefore offers therapists guidelines for

■ Active engagement of the client in the therapy process, promoting an understanding of his/her position within a journey towards a desired state.
■ Active management of the therapist's own role – alternating between leading and following within the therapy situation.

Applied to vocational rehabilitation, these guidelines are particularly helpful when considering a starting point for intervention, matched to the client's motivation, and to ensure that grading and review takes place throughout the intervention and integration into society remains the end goal. Du Toit commented

> *work preparation must lead to reality and not to a sentimental nothingness, nor to accumulate non-functional physical capacities. It must prepare him to fulfil a real role in life, a role compatible with his intellectual, physical and personality abilities… (Du Toit, 1968, p.7).*

Using the model can increase therapists' confidence when having to make decisions around engaging with vocational work themselves, or when they have to guide others in the employment team to understand the needs of their clients.

Case studies

To illustrate the use of the concepts described, two cases are used, one from South Africa and the other from England.

Case Study 10.1   Joe

Joe was 18 years old. He was poorly educated and lived with his parents on a farm in a very rural part of South Africa, where his father was a labourer. He was admitted to a mental health unit because of an acute episode of psychosis induced by excessive smoking of cannabis. He lived far away from medical attention and was surprised to learn that smoking cannabis could have the effects on him that it had. Joe helped his father with tasks on the farm and around the house and he managed to survive as his parents took care of his basic needs, but there was no money for extras. He met a woman shortly before becoming unwell and was concerned that she would not want any more to do with him because of his behaviour when he was psychotic.

Although his formal education was limited, Joe was quick witted and understood a great deal about social discrimination, the stigma of mental illness and how this could impact on his future. He felt afraid and hopeless, resulting in a depressed mood. He had a good understanding and a keen interest in farming practices, although his farm work was unpaid. He also enjoyed general do-it-yourself work around the house and was very skilled in various aspects of building, plastering, painting and decorating. He hoped that he would eventually be offered a paid job by the farmer and was therefore motivated to show how hard he could work. Unfortunately, the farmer was aware of Joe's episode of mental illness and asked his father to make sure that he did not return as he did not want to be responsible for his actions should he become unwell on the farm.

(Continued)

Case Study 10.1 *Continued*

Joe was heartbroken by this news, and it was difficult to engage him in thinking about a future. In terms of his level of creative ability, he functioned on passive participation – the therapist-directed phase. This meant that Joe had a consolidated task concept, and presented as compliant and conforming to social norms. At this level, it was important for the occupational therapist to offer structure to Joe's day, leading him in activities that would interest him and gradually withdrawing support in order for him to become more self-directed. Identifying different pathways towards work helped Joe to recognise where most of his productive activities were centred and in which work sector he ultimately wanted to be employed. Although the future initially looked bleak for Joe, with no formal record of employment, poor education and high unemployment figures in the area, there were many initiatives, around the end of the apartheid era, for young black men to be empowered. After talking to the farmer about a reference for the work that Joe had done on the farm, the occupational therapist helped Joe to apply for funding to set up a smallholding, growing apples. The funding included training in entrepreneurship to assist with financial management. Although the funding application was not fully successful, Joe was offered a place on the entrepreneurial course. This was an ideal situation, as it matched his interests and challenged him just enough to encourage creative effort. As a result, Joe excelled on the course and the trainers became aware of his other skills.

Then, he had started to frame his previous work differently. He called it work experience and voluntary work, validating what he had been involved in, rather than considering himself and his efforts as unworthy due to lack of payment for what he had done. Joe was offered a voluntary position with the college as a fieldwork assistant to the lecturer in agricultural studies. He had achieved a sense of pride and this role, and working alongside other students, gave him the confidence to further his own education. The last contact with him indicated that Joe was still at the college, studying for a certificate in education whilst being offered a temporary paid job using his painting and decorating skills, alongside being a fieldwork assistant. His experience of mental illness exposed him to a different way of thinking about himself, and he managed to overcome the many potential obstacles towards being employed in the sector he wanted to be. His journey, however, shows that vocational goals are dynamic and fluid, with movement between employment sectors leading on to new thinking and decision making.

Case Study 10.2 Janet

Janet was referred to a community mental health team with a diagnosis of generalised anxiety disorder. She experienced panic attacks, and at the time of her referral, was reluctant to go out of her house. She was in her late thirties, married with two teenaged children. She was a caring mother and close to her family. Her sister accompanied her to the initial assessment. Janet's anxiety started when she was verbally abused by a group of teenagers while at work in the local newsagent where she was employed until three o'clock every day, when she left to pick up her own children from school. The abuse started when Janet asked the group for identification to sell alcohol to them and they refused. They were at the shop every morning when Janet arrived to open it and they shouted abuse at her. Janet's managers were supportive of her, but did not change her duties. They felt that it would soon blow over. Although they were correct and it did, Janet started feeling anxious and depressed and could not return to work. The family relied on her income and her time off work caused a great deal of stress when her salary was eventually reduced due her time off work.

(Continued)

Case Study 10.2   *Continued*

Janet's level of creative ability at the time of assessment was self-presentation, self-directed phase. Her actions were explorative as she was searching for meaning in her life and trying to make sense of what had happened to her. Few of her efforts were sustained and she became absorbed in thinking about her fears. She was ego-centric and unable to appreciate the needs of others. As she functioned on a higher level before, she was very aware of her creative capacity, and this conflict caused her to feel guilty and worthless.

At this level, it was important for Janet and her occupational therapist to allow time for exploration of her feelings. A discussion around the different work sectors, described earlier, facilitated such an exploration well as it linked in with her dilemma around having a vocational goal. Once Janet understood that her daily activities constituted work in different sectors of society, she realised that most of her productive energy was spent around her house and in caring for others. Even though she was unable to fulfil her obligations as a paid worker, she was involved in caring for her elderly father through doing his shopping and household management. In exploring this further, Janet mentioned that, as a child, she had cared for her grandmother and that she started some nursing training before she was married. Although she had worked at the newsagent for several years, she viewed it as convenient but not something she found stimulating or particularly enjoyable. She also recognised that her anxiety was particular to the job, the events surrounding it and the financial concerns should she not return. Janet now formulated her vocational goal, still in the paid, public sector, but she decided to contact a care agency to explore her options rather than return to her previous role. She discovered that carers were in demand and that she could specify the hours that she wanted to work. She also had a bigger earning potential in the field. Janet decided to resign from her job at the newsagent when she was offered a part-time caring job. She went from strength to strength once she worked her first shift. Her caring nature and the job she was doing were well matched. She received good feedback from her employers, and her confidence increased. She has since taken up nursing again through an initiative to have previously trained nurses return to practice, and feels that she has finally fulfilled her potential.

Summary

In this chapter, I have shared several influences on my career as an occupational therapist in mental health. My journey started in a general hospital, and this has illustrated how an interest in the totality of human experience helped to shape my understanding of mental health. A theme throughout my story, and evident in my work, is that the concept of health is a dynamic state on a continuum, and that anyone, at any particular time, could be at any point on it. This assumption draws me to use models and approaches, which reflects the dynamic nature of a state of health and assists my understanding of the narratives of the people I work with. I have focused on how occupational therapy may contribute to employment and vocational services from a profession-specific perspective when introducing the model of creative ability (Du Toit, 1972) and covered how a classification of work in society (Taylor, 2003) could be used to identify vocational goals and outcomes.

I also offered some information on the context in which employment services are being developed for mental health service users in England, and how this work reflects the need for individual and holistic regard of the person's narrative to meet vocational goals and aspirations.

Questioning your Practice

1. Which core concepts of occupational therapy can be extracted from the author's account of her career?
2. How do occupational therapists position themselves in the field of employment and vocational opportunities? What is their unique contribution/perspective in this field?
3. How could different cultural contexts and political drivers impact clients and practitioners of employment and vocational issues for persons suffering with mental health problems?

References

Bond GR (2004) Supported employment: evidence for evidence-based practice. *Psychiatric Rehabilitation Journal, 27(4)*, 345–359.

Crowther R, Marshall M, Bond G, Huxley P (2001) *Vocational Rehabilitation for People with Severe Mental Illness.* The Cochrane Database of Systematic Reviews (2) Art. No : CD 003080. DOI: 10.1002/14651858.

Colson A, Howells L (2005) *Routes2Employment – Positive about Mental Health,* London: ELCMHT; NELMHT.

Creek J (2003) *Occupational Therapy Defined as a Complex Intervention,* London: College of Occupational Therapists.

De Witt PA (2005) Creative ability: a model for psychosocial occupational therapy. In: R Crouch, V Alers (eds) *Occupational Therapy in Psychiatry and Mental Health.* London: Whurr Publishers Ltd, 3–61.

Department of Health (2000a) *The NHS Plan.* London: Stationery Office.

Department of Health (2000b) *Meeting the Challenge: A Strategy for the Allied Health Professions.* London: DoH.

Department of Health (2001) *Arrangements for consultant posts for staff covered by the professions allied to medicine PT "A" Whitley Council: Pay for 2001/2002.* London: DoH.

Du Toit V (1968) *A Technique for the Early Introduction of a Work-Related Occupational Therapy Program for the Patient Who Will Retain Significant Residual Disability.* Pretoria: Pretoria College of Occupational Therapy.

Du Toit V (1972) The restoration of activity participation leading to work participation. *South African Journal of Occupational Therapy (2)*, 6–10.

Du Toit V (1974) An investigation into the correlation between volition and its expression. *South African Journal of Occupational Therapy,* 6–10.

Du Toit V (1991) *Patient Volition and Action in Occupational Therapy.* (2nd edn). South Africa: The Vona and Marie du Toit Foundation.

Glucksmann M (1995) Why work? Gender and the total social organisation of labour. *Gender, Work and Organisation, 2(2)*, 63–75.

Mahler J, Tavano S, Gerard C, Baber P (2001) *The Recovery Model: A Conceptual Framework and Implementation Plan.* Contra Costa County Mental Health Recovery Task Force, 1–8.

National Social Inclusion Programme (2005) *First Annual Report.* London: CSIP/NIMHE.

National Social Inclusion Programme (2006) *Vocational Services for People with Severe Mental Health Problems: Commissioning Guidance.* London: DWP/DoH/CSIP.

Office of the Deputy Prime Minister (2004) *Social Exclusion Unit Report: Mental Health and Social Exclusion.* London: ODPM.

Prime Minister's Strategy Unit (2005) *Improving the Life Chances of Disabled People.* London: Cabinet Office.

Taylor R (2003) Extending conceptual boundaries: work, voluntary work and employment. *Work, Employment and Society, 18(1),* 29–49. Cambridge: Cambridge University Press.

11 Powerful stories and challenging messages

Graeme Smith

Personal narrative

It was Monday 10 December 1980, 5 days before my fourteenth birthday when I first experienced what I called a *'fright night'*. Often when my mother, stepfather, two brothers and younger sister went to bed, I would sneak downstairs and get my supplies of glue, lighter fluid and cannabis. This time I added cocaine and went to my stepfather's greenhouse. He grew prize leeks and onions; so it was not uncommon for me to be on guard duty against any sabotage from his rivals. A friend joined me, and to this day only he and I know his identity. This time it was different: it may have been the excitement of my birthday or that girl at school, with long blonde hair, who had promised to give me 'the best birthday present ever!' After using the cocaine, I started to hear loud noises and voices arguing, led by what I called 'JIM JAM' ranting away; a man's voice (JIM) and the feeling of being in a traffic jam (JAM) unable to escape, so you have to just deal with it. The tomato plants in the greenhouse shrieked at me. My friend told me that I hit him a few times as he tried to talk me down; he finally ran away.

I remember being told to be still and quiet – it felt as though the ground had shackled my feet. I had never been so frightened in my life. I did not know it then, but this was my first psychotic episode. For 3 days, I lived on the streets in my town although my parents thought that I was sleeping at my friend's house. Not only was I petrified that 'JIM JAM' was everywhere, but I was also ashamed, lonely and frightened. Two close friends helped me, and I will always be grateful to them. After the third day the noises and voices calmed down and I convinced myself it had been a bad dream and that it would not happen again.

I returned home the day before my birthday to a cuddle from my mother, who promised a great birthday. But, that night a violent fight broke out between my stepfather and my older brother. I tried to intervene and was hit in the face. My brother left home that night to live with my older sister.

After this, my life changed dramatically and my health suffered badly, leading to endless tests with different doctors. Each time the voices returned, I kept silent: the shame and stigma I felt always overcame the fear and the only way I could deal with it was to sleep. Eventually, I was admitted to hospital where the doctors declared it was a problem with my balance and I had an ear operation. My mother always accompanied me to the doctors and she said, 'if you turn out to be like your uncle Teddy, I will never let you leave us like he had to'. I always felt loved by my mother. Today, I still find my birthday and other family events very difficult; they never live up to my hopes and dreams. Since then 'JIM JAM' has visited me three times: it is still alarming but each time it has been a little easier. Now as a 40 year old I tell people the secret that I have carried around.

This chapter will examine narratives; it will explore mental illness narratives and dominant discourses that prevail in that culture. Transforming narratives will be shared, which illuminate the power of occupation and the apparent simplicity of occupational therapy in bringing about positive change.

Stories inside stories

People tell stories; stories are their identities. Families have stories, which illuminate their history, characteristics and beliefs. Peoples' lives have many stories occurring at the same time, with different stories being told about the same event. No single story can be free of ambiguity or contradiction, nor can it encapsulate or handle all the contingencies of life (Morgan, 2000). I have worked in mental health for nearly 20 years; however, mental health has been a story in my family for much longer. I have written about my uncle Teddy (Smith, 2006) and his 40 years in Winterton Asylum and the impact of 'pathologising' stories on my family. This led to a particular dominant story in our family, *'you must be mad'*.

As occupational therapists, our professional story is full of 'pathologising' language and beliefs that transcend the relationships we try to create with people who use our services. In Teddy's example, narrative ideas were used to co-author an alternative story from *'you must be mad'*. Developing alternative stories is a way of responding to these dominant narratives, and this is congruent with the principles of real enablement, valuing people and our interpretations of them. Teddy's alternative story created far more options for understanding him – linked to the lives and values of other people, for example, how madness allowed him to get to the front of a queue by letting his voices out. His paranoia created a wonderful ability to asses risk and manage his loneliness, once telling me that '"*they*" [pointing to his forehead] *are always there and sometimes even they help me'*.

Deconstructing dominant discourses

Working in the context of service user involvement has led me to challenge the notion of power and to question how this influences practice. Dominant stories or discourses in mental health can be deconstructed through therapeutic inquiry. The practices and processes that support suppressive systems or subjugating discourses can be made more visible and thus challenged. These dominant systems tend to exclude service user involvement and, at best, remain tokenistic in fostering service user involvement (King, 2004).

The central role of people in the design and development of the services they use is now recognised (Department of Health, 2001). This chapter aims to assist organisations that are working to involve service users and carers by providing a framework for involvement (Tait & Lester, 2005). It is this process of visibility, transparency and authenticity that needs to be embedded in any structure. This allows service users to step into their power and co-create real changes so that their alternative stories can be listened to and valued. The challenge for occupational therapists is to co-create inclusive practice that is substantive, transformative and valuable to service users and their families.

Narrative examples

In narrative practice, one way of deconstructing dominant and unhelpful stories that people have about their lives is to question the discourses that support these stories. This can assist service users and their families to stop internalising oppressive, marginalising and stigmatising meanings and assumptions, and instead locate these within broader discourses. For example, as a member of a Partnership and Modernisation Board (PAM) multi-agency strategic management group for my organisation, I was asked to develop a service user framework to input into the PAM. A core group, including service users, got together to plan a day to help with this task.

We organised an informal event attended by over 70 service users where we invited stories of disrespectful experiences of involvement. I invited people to imagine disrespect talking, giving us advice about how it thrives, what tricks it gets up to and what would it say. Suddenly the room came alive as individuals gave testimonies about disrespect. I noticed a young man who was wearing a headset. He kept fidgeting and laughing, then he sat silently for about 10 minutes. I returned my attention to the rest of the group and we began discussing what is helpful or unhelpful when he held up his hand and pointed to the headset; I asked if he wanted to speak, and he just pointed again. Then another man said *'he is telling you that the headset lets him speak and listen to his voices'*. I thought what wonderful creativity; the headset helped him contribute to the discussion.

Resulting from this, part of our service user involvement strategy was to provide headsets; this young man is now involved in working with other young men, especially from the early intervention psychosis service. We have also established a 'great ideas forum', which pilots such ideas using an evidence-based approach that links into the service user involvement strategy.

afe therapeutic cultures

A safe therapeutic culture is one where occupational therapists have respect and mpathetic recognition for clients' stories. The occupational therapist is responsible for the creation of a space in which the 'not-yet-said' can be said (Goolishan & nderson, 1987), the creation of a safe therapeutic culture (Rober, 1998) in which subjugated or suppressed knowledge can be accessed (White & Epston, 1990). Thus, occupational therapists have to create spaces where clients' stories can emerge; therapists must not overly structure these encounters. This may be difficult, because this space can appear empty, chaotic and risky.

At times this process of giving clients space to tell their story can feel too unsafe and too uncertain, even for the experienced therapist – this is *unsafe uncertainty* (Rober, 1998). At such times occupational therapists may retreat temporarily to a safer space taking a technical-rational approach or being the expert. When therapists revert to disease pathology to guide their thinking and judgement, this can be considered as an issue of power and they should seek to return to listening to their clients' stories to create a new position of safe uncertainty (Rober, 1998; Smith, 2006). This way of working may be at variance with the multi-disciplinary team, who feel more comfortable with the traditional roles.

Professional identity consists of a set of values, attitudes, ideas, knowledge and skills. These combine and meaning is added to them through storylines and story-telling, thus making it possible for practitioners to articulate what is occupational therapy. This is when the process of really listening to the story becomes exciting – hearing occupational therapists speak out. From this perspective, the task of the occupational therapist becomes one of co-authoring within the systems, where they co-exist, allowing a story of professional identity to develop.

Mattingly (1999) suggests that, to develop such an identity, certain skills must be learnt; certain thinking must be completed around clinical reasoning. How we tell our story shapes our practice and the wider profession in relation to current thinking and perspectives.

The development of a professional identity involves fostering narratives consistent with the performance of occupational therapists. There is not one constructed self-contained notion of identity because storying identities are constantly formed in relationships. This is more a constructionist understanding of identity (Shotter & Gergen, 1989). However, occupational therapists can struggle to remove the filter of a model of practice when listening and engaging with a client and can favour the technical-rational story as truth. It is important to believe that it is possible to co-create a context that provides opportunities for the storying of professional identity as this keeps practitioners alert to the moments that can arise for story development: the process of the emancipatory narrative emerging (Smith 2006). For example, Elizabeth Yerxa describes the early struggles of occupational therapy: these stories made the profession stronger and more valued.

Telling stories in ways that make us stronger

I want to tell you about Paul, a 54-year-old married man. He worked as a coalminer and a health-and-safety officer in mines in the north of England, attending to fatal accidents. He described himself as the most frightened man ever, suffering panic attacks and deep bouts of depression. I met him over 10 years ago when he attended a weekly a multi-media/arts group that I set up in a psychiatric day unit. Paul suffered badly from the stigma associated with mental illness and was afraid of anyone finding out he was using mental health services.

Paul's attendance at the weekly group was his only reason for leaving home. He would often just sit and draw a picture or write, saying very little – the stigma had muffled his voice. He would say and do very little in his life; he could not sleep and feared appointments at the out-patient clinic with the consultant psychiatrist. He was afraid of flying and travelling abroad, avoiding any conversation with his family about this.

Although silent in the group, I gradually understood he was really listening, and even with rapid changes in group members, he knew everyone's name. He reminded me who would not be attending, and why, as they all met for refreshments that he organised before and after the group. He began to arrive early to meet new members because he knew what it was like. He started to make signs and labels that would benefit the group; he developed a user-friendly description of the group with quotes from members and worked on the computer to design an evaluation form. This developed into a reflective storied diary, my first real experience of practice that involved narrative and the client's story. Prior to this, the reports to the treatment team were about his anxiety and inability to cope with responsibility or to accept his illness. A narrative about Paul's avoidance behaviour had gained prominence and as result team members talked about referrals to other services.

As he engaged in the group and, in particular, his documentary of himself, some words started to stand out for him, *caring, good advice giver, good listener, trier, polite, clever man*. We began to see a new story being co-created within the group and how he felt the group had helped him. He started to feel different and talked about stories about anti-stigma, stating

> When I come here, it's like there is something in the room, like a feeling I can do all sorts of stuff and it good stuff, and I am acknowledged…like doing the sheets we all fill in. I was amazed at how everybody said it was useful and we help each other…that's what I need…there is no stigma when you say I have this or that (depression)… . I am me and that feels good again… it's like in families like yours Graeme having someone who always pulls you down but then there is your favourite aunt who always reminds you who you are and why she loves you.

He had created this aunt-like narrative because, in his family, like my own, women were strong and fearless. His mother had stopped speaking to him because he had married a woman from a different religion. Using a clever word play, he had started to imagine the story of an aunt, 'anti stigma'. This allowed him and others to see a narrative other than anxiety, and enriching this narrative at home in the family; he imagined 'anti stigma' helping him so that his family saw him as caring and responsible maintaining close relationships with his two married sons. This led him to supporting new group members. He remembered his story of his need to be a strong father and of family life before stigma and anxiety moved in, and I helped him to recruit his occupational activities into his new story to ensure that he could face stigma and anxiety if they returned.

As Paul told his story he noted that his ex-mining-colleagues, who had always valued his opinion and still kept in contact with him, had now revealed that they too were suffering. He described that anxiety and stigma had tricked him into believing he was the only one, and now a new story was emerging that he and others suffering together could also recover together.

He also recalled the strength in his relationship with his wife and that, despite the attempt of anxiety to destroy this, they thrived. As he told the stories of their love, I saw a new strength emerge. I was looking at a different person; it was the way in which he told his story that made him grow stronger and the way that I shared his stories with my colleagues made my practice grow stronger.

The documentation that we developed formed the bulk of the monthly review and ensured that the narrative of occupational therapy became the new resistance against ideas of disease pathology and biomedicine.

Several years later, Paul arrived at my door. 'Now then', he said, 'I managed to move out stigma and anxiety and thanks to you; I now want to be a counsellor'. Paul is now a member of the group of service users who monitor the services I manage. He is now in his final year of a 3-year counselling course, a very proud good father and grandfather, and one who has at least two holidays abroad each year.

The effects of narrative

When we reclaim the stories we want to tell about our lives and when we reconnect with what we have lost or forgotten, then we become stronger. It is important that others bear witness to this process, as it is knowledge in the making. Not only are we telling our stories differently, but we are also listening differently. We are listening for people's abilities, knowledge and skills. Narrative is defined as an account of occurrences Kirkpatrick (1983). Throughout history, stories have passed from generation to generation; they have mystified and healed. Whatever the message for the storyteller and for the listener, the experience of the story connects them to their culture, to their past, to their present and their possible future. During occupational therapy the client and the therapist experience the same story. Sharing the story enables people to understand themselves and the meaning of themselves better (McKay & Ryan, 1995).

We are now finding ways to acknowledge each others' survival stories and to see the abilities that people have by combining the process of the emancipatory narrative and knowledge in the making: this is a powerful formula for co-creating real change in our clients' lives and challenging our practice.

'Stories are not material to be analysed; they are relationships to be entered' Frank (1995, p. 200). Frank's understanding of illness narratives consists of three types: restitution, chaos and quest narratives. The purpose of this classification is not to pre-know or pre-judge (Wungard & Lester, 2001) but to help create knowing by doing and being, by entering into mutual storytelling as a relationship, thus enabling the not knowing position to emerge (Hoffman, 1990). The illness narrative that Frank (1995) calls 'Chaos' brings forth uncertainty as the main plot, where individuals struggle to make sense of their world as the illness narrative takes hold. A Weingarten interpretive 'quest' is to see if something can be learned which is of value to others; leads to new insights; and for the self (Weingarten, 1997, 1999b).

Illness narratives are easily understood, and one of the biggest challenges for occupational therapists is to see their client beyond their illness. The restitution narrative is perhaps the most recognised illness form and the one often encountered by occupational therapists. Here the story focuses on the illness, assessment, treatment and prognosis, but there is little else. It concentrates on ideas relating to the grand narrative of disease pathology of modern medicine, and this is often the only perspective granted any credence. Some people, whose illnesses do not connect with the restitution narrative or who tell their stories in a different way that allows the emancipatory narrative to emerge, may feel disengaged and marginalised by the attention to their illness.

Here, occupational therapy can be at its most powerful. Clients become engaged in occupational therapy when the meanings that they have evolved no longer work for them, for example, at times of stress and crisis. The occupational therapist helps to co-create new meanings that are congruent with the client's context developing knowledge by doing and engaging the client in, and through, meaningful activity. In this manner the client's story is privileged, allowing the client to be heard and their story to unfold.

The essential ingredients of a good story

Peter was 48 years old and had been diagnosed with alcohol problems and depression in 1997. Then 2 years later announced '*I have just got obsessive compulsive disorder*'. He attended the community addiction team (CAT) in the north of England. In the team review meeting I listened to the illness narrative emerge triumphantly, condemning Peter as someone who was manipulative, secretive, incapable of making decisions, difficult to engage, certainly not to be trusted and always late. The restitution illness narrative followed the same story, each time reaching the same conclusions. After a few months he was referred for occupational therapy; I was told not to expect too much but I was a young enthusiastic therapist who believed in hope, and I still do.

After several meetings with Peter, for which he was late but always apologised, he expressed an interest in coming to the twice-weekly men's meal-planning group. He commented 'I make really good Yorkshire puddings; my mother showed us when we were children, and it is all about getting the air in when mixing.' The group met on Tuesdays, when members would plan the meal and allocate tasks, agree on the time that the meal would be cooked and served on Thursday. The group had operated for several weeks but had not yet had a meal cooked and served on time.

During Peter's first group, the eight men agreed that the only way to complete their task was to heat frozen pies and frozen chips. Peter sat and listened to the men deciding where to shop, who would go and how to deal with problems. He interrupted the conversation, 'I can show you all how to make anything you want'. We all looked astonished. 'You see every thing has an essential ingredient especially with cooking, if you remember that ingredient then you are half way there'. He showed the others how to make lists to help remember things, he emphasised the importance of practising and he recalled the way his mother cooked. We began to reminisce about mothers and sons. Suddenly multi-contextual stories emerged. Nine weeks later we sat down together and had served on time a wonderfully cooked Christmas dinner, roast duck with fennel, served with honey roast vegetables and the biggest Yorkshire puddings I had ever seen. The group's favourite saying became – what is the essential ingredient?

An alternative type of expertise had started to emerge. Peter's ability to plan was brilliant, as was the group's capacity to believe in itself when other treatment team members doubted and questioned the group. Over time, Peter's story unfolded and he became the expert because the group created a space for his expertise to come alive. Peter recognised that he had memory problems and asked for tests that later established that he had early-onset dementia. Previously, the narrative of depression and alcohol problems had prevailed. Through the restitution narrative, Peter emerged as a loving father, a humorous, supportive and resourceful friend; his creativity shone through occupational therapy. These stories challenged the dominant narrative and were reported back to the treatment team. Peter later insisted that his key worker put the following on his case notes, 'always wait for Peter because he would always wait for you, and he is the best at being late, something he is very proud of'.

Social inclusion

I reflected with a senior colleague, could occupational therapists today create social inclusion and again become social reformers? The challenge for the profession is to make this happen. We have a responsibility to lead on social reform, as many of our service users experience occupation deprivation. Everyone has a right to participate in occupation and the right to choose not to. My colleague described a wonderful example how to face this challenge.

At lunchtime, Georgina had returned to the ward from attending a creative group in the occupational therapy department where she had been working on one of her paintings of cats. When asked if she would like her lunch she replied, 'I couldn't possibly eat anything; I'm so full of art'. The words 'full of art' are so meaningful, communicating the significance of the activity to her. Her artwork and the group have become part of her identity; her belief is that she is attending art lessons where she excels at painting. This sense of her achievement lasts beyond the sessions and the ward nurses see her work as something to talk about and celebrate. In the ward, she does not respond with much interest to painting and she is unable to concentrate on activities. However, during occupational therapy, she works with precision and her attention can be focused for over half an hour.

Georgina is 82 years old, has led a full and interesting life, but now has Alzheimer's disease. She retains a strong personality but frequently becomes confused and disoriented, paranoid and aggressive towards others. Before she joined the art lessons, staff reported that her mood was low, she isolated herself and would not involve herself in activities. The task for the occupational therapist was to create an environment where Georgina could thrive and where her needs for success, inclusion and identity could be nurtured. Entering into her reality, listening to her thoughts and responding to her humour are more important than the symptoms of her illness.

To make sense of her expression that she could not possibly eat as she was full of art, for me, was the emancipatory narrative, the moment for difference to occur. Bateson (1972) calls this difference that creates a difference. It is the responsibility of the occupational therapist to create enough difference in the story that can allow somebody to be included within their own life to co-create the context where the story can be enriched and others bear witness to this process. Social inclusion becomes part of that process and there is nothing more powerful for individuals, families and communities to feel this. This is where the power is given to the people who need it, when occupational therapy is at it most transformative and occupational therapists become social reformers.

I cannot resist the urge to tell you about people who I work with who inspire me and have helped create knowledge in the making. I am a practitioner who works with clients of all ages in a range of different contexts. I want to finish by coming full circle. I am writing this chapter 12 days before my dreaded birthday. I work in a school in the north with a group of 12–13 year olds children.

I teach part of their personal health social and citizenship education course. In a recent lesson, I was joined by Jean, who told the children a story about her life 3 years ago. She introduced her family through photographs: David, her husband, Mark, her teenage son, Thomas (9) and Jack (6) and their two dogs. They were a family who loved football and having fun.

Jean gave wonderful accounts of intimacy, love and warmth within the family. The children listened carefully – she had their full attention. After 20 minutes she stopped and I asked the children to imagine something that might happen to this family. What would it be? How would life be different? I asked what message would you send that would be helpful to the family. As they discussed in small groups a range of possible stories unfolded:

■ David lost his job because he had depression.
■ Thomas was bullied at school.
■ Mark left home with his girlfriend because she was pregnant.
■ David drank too much and Jean kicked him out.
■ They divorced.

I asked Jean to continue, she slowly rose from her chair, stood silently for a few minutes and then said:

> Mark took his own life about 14 months ago, he hanged himself in our house, in our en suite bedroom…I don't know why, sometimes I think I do but… and I blame myself for not seeing it, you see he seemed happy he was just a normal young lad just like you, he loved his brothers. That day our lives changed forever…I never thought that suicide would be knocking on my door but Graeme has asked me to come today and think that if suicide was to speak what would it say? It would tell you to be quiet, blame yourself, don't tell anyone what is on your mind, everyone is against you, whatever is on your mind or what happens, you are better off not being here…well I think if you feel like Mark might have felt, please talk to someone. It is good to see that these lessons are happening, Mark was your age once and he would have really liked being in a lesson like this.

The children sat spellbound, listening to Jean's every word. I noticed one of the girls scribbling on a piece of paper, and at the end of the lesson the children burst into spontaneous applause for Jean and each in turn thanked her for telling her story. On the way out, the girl handed the paper to me; she had written

> I think Jean is really brave and a lovely mother and she has been through a lot, I think she needs a big hug that is what I would do. The whole family needs a proper massive cuddle. I think that I understand more and that any family like Jean's and mine have to watch out because it can happen to anyone. I loved the lesson, Sir.

Summary

Occupational therapy is a complex intervention (Creek, 2003) and can convey a message of hope, courage and resilience and can co-create a new story connecting the past, present and future. But this can only happen if occupational therapists work across boundaries, believe in themselves, the narrative and the story in the making. We can lead, inspire and find that we have what Peter would call that essential ingredient.

Questioning your practice

1. If good occupational therapy practice could speak, what would *it* say/not say, how would *it* like to be remembered, and what helps *it* thrive, and what do you need to more of to ensure that good occupational therapy survives?
2. Imagine someone close to you in your family using your service; what stories would they tell about their experiences?
3. If there was one thing you could change/have changed in your practice to ensure authentic, meaningful service user involvement, what would it be?

References

Bateson G (1972) *Steps to an Ecology of Mind: Collected Essays in Anthropology, Psychiatry, Evolution, and Epistemology*. Chicago: University Of Chicago Press.

Creek J (2003) *Occupational Therapy as a Complex Intervention*. London: COT Care.

Department of Health (2001) *The Expert Patient: A New Approach to Chronic Disease Management for the 21st Century*. London: HMSO.

Department of Health. http://www.publications.doh. gov.uk/cmo/progress/expertpatient/index. htm. Accessed 12 Feb 2007

Frank AW (1995) *The Wounded Story Teller: Body, Illness, and Ethics*. Chicago, IL: University of Chicago Press.

Goolishan H, Anderson H (1987) Language Systems and Therapy: an evolving idea. *Psychotherapy, 24*, 524–538.

Hoffman L (1990) Constructing realities: an art of lenses. *Family Process, 29(1)*, 1–12.

King S (2004) Commissioned Report on Service User Involvement within the Association of Occupational Therapists in Mental Health. http://www.cot.org.uk/specialist/mentalhealth/intro.php.

Kirkpatrick EM (ed.) (1983) *Chambers 20th Century Dictionary*. London: W&R Chambers.

Mattingly C (1999) *Healing Dramas, Clinical Plots: The Narrative Structure of Experience*. Cambridge, UK: Cambridge University Press.

McKay EA, Ryan S (1995) Clinical reasoning through story telling; examining a student's case story on a fieldwork placement. *British Journal of Occupational Therapy, 58(6)*, 234–238.

Morgan A (2000) What is Narrative Therapy – An Easy Read Introduction. Adelaide, South Australia: Dulwich Centre Publications.

Rober P (1998) Reflections on ways to create a safe therapeutic culture for children in family therapy. *Family Process, 37(2)*, 201–213.

Shotter J, Gergen K (1989) *Texts of Identity*. London: Sage.

Smith G (2006) The Casson Memorial Lecture 2006: Telling tales – how stores and narraive co-create change. *British Journal of Occupational Therapy, 69(7)*, 304–311.

Tait L, Lester H (2005) Encouraging user involvement in mental health services. *Advances in Psychiatric Treatment, 11(3)*, 168–175.

Weingarten K (1997) *The Mothers Voice; Strengthening Intimacy in Families*. (2nd edn). New York Guilford Press.

Weingarten (1999b) *The Politics of Narrative: Who Tells, Who Listens and Who Cares in Narrative Therapy and Community Work; A Conference Collection*. Adelaide: Dulwich Centre publications.

White M, Epston D (1990) *Narrative Means to Therapeutic Ends*. New York: WW Norton.

Wungard B, Lester J (2001) *Telling Our Stories In Ways That Make Us Stronger*. Adelaide, South Australia: Dulwich Centre Publications.

Part III Research and Future Directions

12 Reviewing consumer-run mental health services

Samson Tse and Carolyn Doughty

Personal narratives

Samson Tse

I am an occupational therapist and have always enjoyed working in mental health. I value the interpersonal relationships I have with people and the creative side of working in mental health. I obtained my doctoral degree from the University of Otago, New Zealand. Now I teach at the University of Auckland. My current research includes work on the recovery approach, work rehabilitation, primary health care and mental health. My personal understanding of mental health has shifted in response to years spent in clinical work, reading others' research and conducting my own research. I have moved from concentrating on mental illness or reducing psychiatric disability to focusing on mental health with an emphasis on clients' strengths, resilience, aspirations and goals. After meeting Carolyn Doughty in 2002, I began exploring the topic of peer-support and service-user-led interventions. How do they work? What is the evidence to support this type of service delivery? What are the critical success factors? What are the opportunities and challenges associated with delivering these types of services?

Carolyn Doughty

After working for more than a decade in community mental health, I returned to university to do a PhD in psychological medicine, working with families affected by bipolar disorder. Soon after completion I was employed by a small group of consumers who had a wider vision for growing a network of people within New Zealand that would offer peer support to *tangata whai ora* (those seeking wellness) and their *whanau* (family and significant others). Five years later, this national organisation with grassroots members from across New Zealand continues to grow and develop, linking support groups and peer organisations around the country and seeking to build the capacity of all peer workers in mental health. Since its inception, Balance New Zealand has held highly successful annual training events with a strong emphasis on recovery principles, consumer training and leadership. As an organisation it aims to ensure that any support, information and training provided will be particularly relevant, timely and responsive to consumer needs.

Introduction

Over the last three decades, there have been major shifts in the theoretical paradigm within mental health. The first shift concerned the increasing level of interest in mental health at a population or community level in response to the emerging evidence of very high lifetime prevalence of mental illness in the population particularly in Western countries. The recent Te Rau Hinengaro New Zealand Mental Health Survey (Oakley *et al.*, 2006) estimates that the lifetime risk (up to 75 years of age) of experiencing any common mental disorder such as depression, anxiety or an alcohol or drug disorder is 46.4%. It signals that mental health problems are a concern for the whole population.

The second shift has been the move away from focusing on mental illness to considering mental health, emphasising clients' strengths, resilience, spirituality and aspirations. People with mental health problems recover from mental illness, and they now have the potential to improve the quality of service delivery through active involvement in the mental health system. This may be in a variety of roles such as a consumer consultant or advisor, peer specialist or leading a mental health programme.

Like other health professionals, occupational therapists working in mental health have the opportunity to interact with consumers as colleagues in several ways. This may include work as a paid staff member employed by a consumer-run programme adjunct to a mental health service or working alongside a consumer consultant (Honey, 1999; Corr *et al.*, 2005). Occupational therapists assert that the basic philosophy and value of the profession resonates very strongly with client or consumer-centred practice (Sumsion, 1999; Fossey & Harvey, 2001), but now the challenge and opportunity is to form meaningful alliances with consumers and to work with, and in, consumer-run mental health services. This chapter reviews the literature about consumer-run or consumer-led mental health services and relates observations of the sector. The specific objectives were to

1. Define the terminology and explore issues relevant to consumer-run services.
2. Complete a systematic review to examine the evidence for effectiveness of consumer-run services.
3. Identify some critical success factors and challenges associated with operating consumer-run services.
4. Make recommendations for future research and services development.

Terms and concepts

In this chapter consumers are defined as individuals with mental illness who have been users of mental health services and who identify themselves as such.

The terms service user and consumer are used interchangeably, acknowledging that there is variation in how individuals prefer to be addressed (Mueser *et al.*, 1996). Literature from North America favours the term consumer, while in the UK and Europe service user is in more general use and in New Zealand the Maori term *tangata whai ora* (person seeking wellness) or *tangata motuhake* (another term for people with mental illness) are popular alternatives.

It is not straightforward to define consumer participation or recognise what a consumer-run or consumer-led service is. In Australia, consumer participation in the mental health field has come to mean 'that service providers ensure that consumers have the opportunity to influence decision-making processes in the areas of service delivery, service planning and development, training and evaluation' (Department of Health and Community Services, 1996, p. 5). The operational definition of most consumer-run services (CRS) moves a step beyond what has been described as consumer participation.

It embraces the notion that any support offered, by the CRS, is not controlled or dominated by professionals. This does not necessarily preclude non-consumers or professionals from being involved, but their inclusion is within the control of the consumer operators (Solomon & Draine, 1996). Indeed, it is not uncommon that qualified mental health professionals may have personal experience of mental health problems.

Here, a consumer-run, consumer-led service is defined as a programme, project or service planned, administered, delivered and evaluated by a consumer group based on needs defined by the consumer group. Operation of the service requires consumer self-governance, staffing and supervision of the staff, control of programme policy and responsibility for programme implementation. While there is generally consensus among consumers that staff in traditional mental health services are on the whole well-intentioned, system structures, resource allocation and general attitudinal issues still interact to create barriers for effective service delivery (MacNeil & Abbott, 2000).

Over the last 20 years further effort has been made to empower people with mental illness to increase their activity in and control over mental health services. The notion that consumers can participate and provide useful services to other people has been based on two important foundations. First, mental illness and its associated problems are socially constructed (Hutchison & Pedlar, 1999). Chinman *et al.* (2001, p. 215) argued that a proportion of any individual's ongoing symptoms or psychiatric disability stem from the 'poor person-environment fit between the multiple and complex needs of those with serious psychiatric disorders and community-based mental health systems.' Therefore, consumers working together in service provision are in an ideal position to close the gap between person–environment fit and address the issues faced by their peers on a day-to-day basis such as social isolation, demoralisation, poor quality of life and difficulties in accessing mental health services. Second, because of individuals' personal experience, they are in a unique position to make contributions that will promote positive service development and, therefore, service effectiveness by improving outcomes for mental health clients.

The potential benefits of intentional peer support include, but are not limited to, sharing similar life experiences in making sense of mental illness-related experiences, regaining a sense of control that counteracts feelings of powerlessness, role modelling recovery, instillation of hope, providing more empathetic and relevant emotional support, sharing practical information and coping strategies and strengthening social supports (Felton, *et al.*, 1995; Mowbray *et al.*, 2005). Consumers, as mental health service providers, are sometimes seen as more sensitive, as they more readily see the person rather than the illness. Employing service users within clinical settings or using consumer organisations as providers can facilitate cultural change within mental health workplaces by stimulating open dialogue on the attitude and behaviours of professionals. It breaks down stigma and promotes a vision of inclusion and the full participation of service users in society. It demonstrates that mental health services value consumer experience if they also employ them in providing services to others (Solomon & Draine, 1996). Lastly, CRSs or consultants can work towards social justice and enduring social change on behalf of individuals with mental illness (Mowbray *et al.*, 2005).

CRSs can be divided into three main categories (Clay, 2005). The first, drop-in centres, are places where members can meet in a relaxing manner and participate in activities of their choice. The second, peer support programmes, provide a unique opportunity for individuals in recovery to support one another. The final, education programmes, consist of small groups in which participants learn about recovery, relapse prevention or stress-coping skills. Additional ways in which consumer involvement is possible in both partnership services or consumer-run or consumer-operated services are summarised in Box 12.1.

Despite the claims made about the desirability of consumers' involvement, it remains a challenge to define what is meant by involving consumers in mental

---

Box 12.1 Ways in which consumers can be involved in mental health services, modified from the work by Simpson and House (2002, 2003).

Current or former consumer	Qualified clinical staff with personal experience of mental health problems
	Provider in traditional mental health services, e.g., peer specialist on case management team or crisis team, mental health support worker or consumer advisor along with clinical staff
	Provider of independent mental health services, e.g., a consumer consultant providing information and advocacy services
	Trainer of mental health service providers/family or carers/other consumers or students, e.g., health professional training, health professionals' ongoing education, intentional peer support or self management/recovery training
	Research, audit or evaluation of mental health services
	Advisors in public policy and programme development

Adapted and reproduced with permission from the *BMJ* Publishing Group's *British Medical Journal*, 325, 1265.

health services and to embed this in practice. Information on the strength of evidence about the effectiveness of consumer operated services and programmes could add value to existing mental health services in countries currently struggling with this issue, such as the US, Canada, the UK, Australia and New Zealand.

Reviewing effectiveness of consumer-run services

Methodology

A systematic method of literature searching and selection was employed. Searches were limited to English language material published from 1980 to May 2004. Peer-reviewed studies were considered if they used one of the following study designs: systematic review, randomised controlled trials (including cross-over trials), pseudo-randomised controlled trials (alternate allocation or some other method), concurrent controls or cohort studies, case-control studies, cross-sectional or descriptive studies. Evidence, obtained from case studies without outcome data, was excluded, but these may be used as examples in the discussion. Descriptive studies, where there was no control group, were included and described but not tabled. Key outcome measures for primary studies related to the effectiveness of relevant interventions included, but not limited to, improved income, level of functioning, quality of life, attitudes to use of medication, social contacts, symptoms, inpatient days, clients' satisfaction or perception of the service, hospital admissions, nature or duration of hospitalisations, time until first hospitalisation, arrest, emergency hospital care or homelessness, use of crisis services, self-esteem, engagement in programme, employment and relationship between client and case manager.

Studies were selected for appraisal using a two-stage process. Initially, the titles and abstracts (where available) were identified from the search strategy, including references cited in retrieved papers and review articles; these were scanned and excluded as appropriate. The full text articles were retrieved for the remaining studies and these were appraised if they fulfilled the following study inclusion and exclusion criteria (Table 12.1).

The strength of the evidence in the selected studies was assessed and classified using the dimensions of evidence defined by the National Health and Medical Research Council, Canberra, Australia. These are derived directly from the literature identified as informing a particular intervention. The designations of the levels of evidence are shown in Table 12.2 and the three subdomains (level, quality and statistical precision) are collectively a measure of the strength of the evidence (National Health and Medical Research Council, 2000).

Results

Studies included in the review

The search strategy identified over 175 studies. After excluding studies from the search titles, abstracts and reference lists, 85 full text articles were retrieved, of these 57 did not fulfil the inclusion criteria and were excluded. The remaining 28

Table 12.1 Inclusion/exclusion criteria for identification of relevant studies.

Characteristic	Criteria
Inclusion criteria	
Publication type	Studies published 1980 or later
Sample characteristics	Adults (aged 18 years or more)
	Study population those with Axis I psychiatric disorders as classified by DSM-IV and/or ICD-10 or earlier versions of these classifications
	Studies that were not restricted to participants within these age ranges, but met any of the following criteria: results were reported separately on a subgroup of participants aged at least 13 years of age; the mean age for the sample was at least 13 years
Sample size	Studies with sample size 5 or more people
Intervention/test	Consumer-run or consumer-led mental health services for people with mental disorders
	Comparative or controlled studies of consumer participation services within mental health services where led by consumer steering group, managed, implemented or staffed primarily by consumers
Comparators	Traditional health professional-run and/or directed mental health services
Outcome	Studies using at least one outcome measure examining the effectiveness of the intervention in achieving improvement in function or quality of life for consumers using the service, studies looking at service delivery or studies looking at indirect measures of effectiveness
Exclusion criteria	
Publication type	Non-systematic reviews, letters, editorials, expert opinion articles, comments, book chapters, articles published in abstract form and studies on animal subjects
	Non-published work
Language	Non-English language articles will be excluded
Study design	Evidence obtained from case studies/series where there is no outcome data
Sample	Studies which report outcomes for a study population including 50% or more with DSM IV alcohol or drug abuse and/or dependence as the presenting diagnosis will be excluded
	Studies which primarily concern participants with physical or neurological conditions such as multiple sclerosis
Intervention/test	Studies investigating consumer involvement in mental health services but where health professionals retain 50% or more of the role of governance or management of the specific service or event (not including overall governance of the wider mental health service within which an initiative might be placed)
Outcome	Studies which used no quantitative outcome measure or proxy measure for collecting and reporting data from study participants

Table 12.2 Explanation of the levels of evidence and strength of evidence (National Health and Medical Research Council, 2000).

Level of evidence	Study design
I	Evidence obtained from a systematic review of all relevant randomised controlled trials
II	Evidence obtained from at least one properly-designed randomised controlled trial
III-1	Evidence obtained from well-designed pseudo-randomised controlled trials (alternate allocation or some other method)
III-2	Evidence obtained from comparative studies (including systematic reviews of such studies) with concurrent controls and allocation, not randomised, cohort studies, case–control studies or interrupted time series with a control group
III-3	Evidence obtained from comparative studies with historical control, two or more single arm studies, or interrupted time series without a parallel control group
IV	Evidence obtained from case series, either post-test or pre-test/post-test

Strength of evidence	Definition
Level	The study design used, as an indicator of the degree to which bias has been eliminated by design
Quality	The methods used by investigators to minimise bias within a study design
Statistical precision	The p-value or, alternatively, the precision of the estimate of the effect. It reflects the degree of certainty about the existence of a true effect

articles were eligible for inclusion and were fully appraised, consisting of 26 papers reporting primary research and 2 papers reporting systematic reviews, which will be discussed next.

Davidson and colleagues (1999) provided a valuable commentary on the historical development and potential effectiveness of peer support among individuals with serious mental illness. Their review focused on naturally occurring mutual support groups, consumer-run services and employment of consumers as health providers. Most studies included in this review were descriptive, were limited by their small samples and low power and did not have random assignment. A more recent systematic review (Simpson and House, 2002) considered the evidence involving users in the delivery and evaluation of mental health services. This comprehensive review was based on research published between 1966 and 2001, and included randomised controlled trials and comparative studies.

The remaining 26 eligible primary research studies included 6 randomised controlled trials (Solomon & Draine, 1996; Klein, Cnaan & Whitecraft, 1998; Clark *et al.*, 1999; O'Donnell *et al.*, 1999; Paulson*et al.*, 1999; Campbell, 2004); 7 comparative studies (Polowczyk *et al.*, 1993; Cook *et al.*, 1995; Felton *et al.*, 1995; Lyons*et al.*, 1996;

Chinman *et al.*, 2000; Chinman *et al.*, 2001; Segal & Silverman, 2002) and 13 descriptive studies (Chen, 1990; Mowbray & Tan, 1993; Chamberlin *et al.*, 1996; Segal*et al.*, 1997; Torrey *et al.*, 1998; Hutchison & Pedlar, 1999; Bentley, 2000; Petr *et al.*, 2000; Segal *et al.*, 2000; Meehan *et al.*, 2002; Mowbray,*et al.*, 2002; Salzer & Shear, 2002; Tobin *et al.*, 2002) identified for appraisal from the search strategy.

A variety of interventions were considered. These included the involvement of current or former users of mental health services as providers in mental health services, for example, as case managers in a community mental health service (Solomon & Draine, 1996), case managers in an assertive community treatment programme (Paulson *et al.*, 1999), client consumer advocates attached to a case management service (O'Donnell *et al.*, 1999), peer counsellors alongside a case management service (Klein *et al.*, 1998); peer specialists on case management teams (Felton *et al.*, 1995), case managers in outreach service (Chinman *et al.*, 2000), service providers in a community outreach service (Chinman *et al.*, 2001) and users as service providers in a mobile crisis assessment service (Lyons *et al.*, 1996). One study looked at current or former users of mental health services as trainers of mental health service providers (Cook *et al.*, 1995). All these studies were published between 1993 and 2002, and these proximal publication dates indicate the relatively recent development of this field of enquiry. One unpublished randomised trial was included because of its significance for the field (Campbell, 2004).

Nineteen out of twenty-six of the evaluations to date appear to have been conducted in the US (76%). Notably, three studies from Australia (12%) have been included, two from Canada (8%) and one from the UK (4%). No published New-Zealand-based studies or evaluations were identified from the search strategy used regardless of study design.

All the Level I, II and III studies included in this review are presented in Table 12.3, using the terminology and spelling of the country of origin.

Summary of evidence

Most research in mental health draws on three major types of studies: true experiments, quasi-experiments and case–control designs. Given the limited level of knowledge in regard to self-help and consumer-operated programmes, it is appropriate to also use non-controlled study designs (Mowbray & Tan, 1993). Unlike the work by Davidson and colleagues (1999), the recent review by Simpson and House (2002) only considered controlled or comparative study designs, namely, randomised controlled trials as these are considered the gold standard for evaluating effectiveness. However, Chen (1990) asserts that evaluators should first address whether programmes are serving their targeted beneficiaries, with service delivery activities and programmes as intended, and meeting their specified objectives. Once this is assured, experimental designs for outcome evaluation may be considered, but not before. Otherwise, it cannot be known whether unsuccessful outcomes reflect failure of the specified model or failure to implement the model as specified. For this reason, selected high-quality descriptive studies were also included in this review. The following three sections discuss the literature appraised.

Table 12.3 Summary of Level I, II and III studies on the effectiveness of consumer-run or consumer-led mental health services.

Source	Level of evidence, Design, Objective and Methods	Results and Original Authors' Conclusions
Davidson et al. (1999) Clinical Psychology: Science and practice	Secondary research, level I; systematic review, USA Reviewed historical development and potential effectiveness of peer support among persons with severe mental illness. The three primary modes of peer support included in this review were: (1) naturally occurring mutual support groups, (2) consumer-run services and (3) employment of consumers as providers within mental health services.	Regarding naturally occurring mutual support groups, the evidences on effectiveness remain tentative. It seems to help social integration among individuals with mental health problems. It was suggested that mutual support groups should focus on supporting mental health treatment, addressing mental health concerns and engage large number of individuals particularly in non-group settings given the low utilisation and high drop put rates Regarding consumer run services, it was suggested that consumer-run services can provide useful services and a constructive peer role model for those recovering from mental illness. The services tend to have strong minority representations. Service-user-run services might be more sensitive to issues of discrimination against people with mental illness and cultural minority background Regarding consumers as service providers or health professionals, it consistently showed that service users can adequately provide services to others with serious mental illness
Simpson & House (2002) British Medical Journal	Secondary research, level I; systematic review, UK It aimed to identify evidence from comparative studies on the effects of involving users in the delivery and evaluation of mental health services.	Five randomised controlled trials and seven comparative studies were identified. Half of the studies considered involving users in managing cases. Involving users as employees of mental health services led to clients having greater satisfaction with personal circumstances and less hospitalisation Mental health service users can be involved as employees, trainers, or researchers without detrimental effect. Involving mental health service users with severe mental disorders in the delivery and evaluation of services is feasible

(Continued)

Table 12.3 Continued

Source	Level of evidence, Design, Objective and Methods	Results and Original Authors' Conclusions
Campbell (2004) Overview and preliminary Findings (Research Report)	Primary study, level II; randomised controlled trial, USA This preliminary report provided the rationale, methods, participants baseline characteristics, and selected outcome findings of a bigger randomised controlled study, Consumer-Operated Service Program Multisite Research Initiative. The experimental conditions consisted of consumer-operated services programmes offered as adjunct to traditional mental health services and the control condition consisted of traditional mental health services. This project involved four drop-in centers, two mutual support programmes and two educational programmes. 1827 participants with severe and persistent mental illness were assessed at baseline, 4, 8 and 12 months measuring 'well-being'. A fidelity assessment tool was developed and used to measure programme characteristics and programme cost	The preliminary findings of the 12-month follow-up study were: (1) both experimental and controlled groups showed improved well-being over time; (2) Further analysis indicated that participants randomly assigned to consumer-operated services programmes of drop-in centers in addition to traditional mental health services showed greater improvement in well-being over the course of study than participants randomly assigned to only traditional mental health services at those sites. However this preliminary study did not evaluate the degree and timing of participation in the services programmes

Clark *et al.* (1999) Psychiatric Services	Primary study, level II; randomised controlled trial, Canada A study at two outpatient facilities compared two methods of collecting data on client satisfaction with mental health services provided by case managers and by physicians. A satisfaction survey instrument was developed with input from clients. A total of 120 clients were randomly assigned to be interviewed by either a staff member or a client	No difference between the two groups was found in overall satisfaction with services received from case managers or physicians. Clients from both facilities reported high levels of satisfaction regardless of the type of interviewer. Clients interviewed by the client interviewers had been ill for a longer period of time than those interviewed by staff members (*p*<.02). The other variables examined were age, number of admissions, gender, marital status, education level and frequency of visitors to the facility. Clients from both facilities reported high levels of satisfaction regardless of the interviewer but clients give more negative responses when interviewed by clients
O'Donnell *et al.* (1999) Australian and New Zealand Journal of Psychiatry	Primary study, level II; randomised controlled trial, Australia This study investigated the provision of client-focused services to community-based clients with schizophrenia and bipolar disorder. It hypothesised that the delivery of more client-focused services would improve client outcome in terms of functioning, disability and satisfaction with services. Clients referred for case management were randomly allocated to one of three groups: standard case management (*n*=35), client-focused case management (*n*=39), or client-focused case management plus consumer advocacy (*n*=45)	While there were no differences between the groups on quantitative measures of functioning, disability, quality of life, service satisfaction and burden of care, there were significant between-group differences on qualitative measures of satisfaction with services. Several methodological difficulties hampered the interpretation of findings. Although clients did not differ on outcome measures of functioning and disability, the group receiving client-focused case management reported greater satisfaction with service delivery

(Continued)

Table 12.3 Continued

Source	Level of evidence, Design, Objective and Methods	Results and Original Authors' Conclusions
Paulson *et al.* (1999) Community Mental Health Journal	Primary study, level II; randomised controlled trial, USA The practice patterns of consumer and non-consumer providers of assertive community treatment were compared using both quantitative and qualitative data collected as part of a randomised trial. This study sought to determine whether the teams differed in the type and amount of time spent on each of tasks performed	The activity log shows that case managers performed a mix of both direct service and administrative tasks. Overall only minor differences were found in the distribution of time spent on various case manager activities. Both teams spent the majority of time providing support and structure (14% consumer, 15% non-consumer), and coordinating services (8%, 8% respectively). Case managers spent approximately one-third of their time with clients with no difference between teams in the amount of time spent face-to-face or on the telephone. One quarter of the time was spent alone and the remaining time (6%) with family members, staff at other agencies and residential operators The qualitative data revealed that there were discernible differences in the 'culture' of the two teams. The consumer team 'culture' emphasised 'being there' with the client while the non-consumer team was more concerned with accomplishing tasks
Klein et al. (1998) Research on Social Work Practice	Primary study, level II; randomised controlled trial, USA The aim of this study was to examine a peer social support programme to high risk dually diagnosed clients. The key research question was whether intensive case management (ICM) coupled with peer support (Friends Connection) would provide: (a) a more cost effective approach to quality service, and (b) significantly affect system outcomes and client integration into the community. A pilot study of 10 randomly selected clients in the study group, and 51 in the comparison group, who had been in community care 1 year prior to this investigation was carried out. Service was provided for a 6-month period	The number of crisis events of the comparison group far exceeded that of the study group. Crisis events included suicide attempts, disturbances in the place of residence, and attacks on staff that necessitated special intervention by agency staff. The number of hospitalisations was dramatically reduced. Clients in the study group reported improved quality of life and perceived their physical and emotional wellbeing as improved over the course of the study Findings suggest that coupling peer social support with intensive case management is associated with positive system outcomes

| Solomon & Draine (1996) Research on Social Work and Practice | Primary study, level II; randomised controlled trial, USA
This study examined whether a team of mental health consumers delivered intensive case management services differently than a team of non-consumer case managers
96 seriously mentally ill clients were randomly assigned to consumer and non-consumer teams of case managers. Teams received the same training, continuing education, and mental health systems support | 91 clients stayed in study. Although there were no differences in total service units between teams, the teams differed in terms of location, manner, and with whom the service was delivered. Consumer managers delivered more services face-to-face with the client and fewer services in the office and in interactions with family members and other mental health service providers
This study supports the contention that consumers can provide client-centered and service-oriented case management services using a service planning and monitoring model. This study did not address whether they could provide a clinical case management model |
| Chinman et al. (2001) Community Mental Health Journal | Primary study, level III; comparative study, USA
This study described the Welcome Basket Program (WBP) and reported preliminary outcome data from a pilot study to evaluate its effectiveness. WBP is an outreach and engagement programme developed, staffed and managed entirely by mental health consumers
WBP participants who also were receiving outpatient services at the centre (the intervention) were compared with a matched sample of people receiving outpatient services at the centre only (standard care condition) | 92 people received outpatient services at the centre. Of these only 14 (15%) were readmitted to hospital, which was a 50% reduction in re-hospitalisations compared with the general outpatient population.
The data suggests that WBP clients were initially at greater risk for re-hospitalisation, and that WBP intervention showed promise in reducing hospitalisation rates among a population at risk |

(Continued)

Table 12.3 Continued

Source	Level of evidence, Design, Objective and Methods	Results and Original Authors' Conclusions
Chinman *et al.* (2000) Journal of Nervous and Mental Disease	Primary study, level III; comparative study, USA This study compared the outcomes of services provided by case managers who were mental health system consumers and case managers who were not consumers Overall sample size for non-consumer sites (*n*=1985), with a mean age 38.52 years; for consumer sites (*n*=950), with a mean age 38.27 years. Number of users involved not specifically stated. Inclusion criterion was prior psychiatric treatment	Although there were significant effects of Time for almost every outcome measure (e.g. clients improved over time) there were no significant Time × Case Manager interactions. Staff age, race, or gender did not significantly alter the pattern of these results Given that services provided by consumers and non-consumers were associated with equivalent outcomes, the present study showed, using a large sample, the ability of consumers to provide mental health services as members of a case management team
Cook *et al.* (1995) Community Mental Health Journal	Primary study, level III; comparative study, USA This project used a randomised design to test the effects of using consumers as trainers for mental health service providers 57 mental health professionals (mean age 34.5 years) participated in a two-day training designed to acquaint trainees with the attitudes and knowledge necessary for delivering 'assertive case management' services Participants were randomly assigned to one of two conditions: one in which they received the second day of training from a consumer and the other involving training by a non-consumer.	Analyses revealed that post-training attitudes were significantly more positive for those participants trained by the consumer. Subjective evaluations also reflected positive reactions to the use of consumers as trainers. Even controlling for pre-test attitudes and respondent background characteristics, those in the experimental condition showed more positive post-test attitudes overall, and felt more positively about consumers as service providers and trainers, and expressed more non-stigmatising attitudes than those trained solely by the non-consumer The use of a consumer trainer achieved positive results and enhanced the effectiveness of the training. If the goal is to make mental health service delivery training an insightful and integrative experience, this study provides preliminary evidence that this type of approach is viable

Felton et al. (1995) Psychiatric Services	Primary study, level III; comparative study, USA A quasi-experimental, longitudinal, non-equivalent control group design was used to compare outcomes of clients assigned to three case management conditions: teams of case managers plus peer specialists, teams of case managers plus non-consumer assistants, and case managers only	Complete data was available for 104 clients. Compared with clients in the other two groups, clients served by teams with peer specialists demonstrated greater gains in several areas of quality of life and an overall reduction in the number of major life problems experienced. They also reported more frequent contact with their case managers and the largest gains of all three groups in the area of self-image and outlook and social support. No statistically significant differences in outcomes were found between clients served by teams with non-consumer assistants and those served by case managers only. However, effect size comparisons showed that clients in the peer specialist group posted the largest gains on 20 of 31 measures
Lyons et al. (1996) Community Mental Health Journal	Primary study, level III; comparative study, USA This study investigated consumer service delivery in a mobile assessment programme designed to assist homeless people with severe psychiatric disorders The programme was designed to serve people both mentally ill and homeless, on a 16-h basis. Staff with prior consumer experience were hired.	Consumer and non-consumer dyads of staff were generally comparable. Results suggested that consumer staff were engaged in more street outreach ($p<.001$) and were less often dispatched for emergencies ($p<.01$). There was a trend for consumer staff to be more likely to certify their clients for psychiatric hospitalisation ($p<.05$) Consumer staff appeared to provide a valuable contribution to this form of service delivery. Mobile assessment staff with personal consumer experience was more likely to do street outreach than were non-consumer staff. This is consistent with the hypothesis that consumer staff were more willing and better able to engage mentally ill people on the street. Several consumer staff chose to communicate their own experiences to the clients they were serving on the street
Polowczyk et al. (1993) Hospital & Community Psychiatry	Primary study, level III; comparative study, USA Examined the use of consumer interviewers (n=225) and staff interviewers (n=305)	Group comparisons revealed no significant differences in age or other demographic characteristics Patients surveyed by both groups of surveyors reported a high level of satisfaction with outpatient services. The mean satisfaction scores were significantly lower in the patient surveyed group ($p<.05$). However, 95% of patients surveyed by staff responded positively compared to 90% of those surveyed by patients

(Continued)

Table 12.3 Continued

Source	Level of evidence, Design, Objective and Methods	Results and Original Authors' Conclusions
Polowczyk et al. (1993) Hospital & Community Psychiatry	Subjects were 530 individuals with serious and persistent mental illness who were attending ten outpatient clinics, three continuing treatment centers, and a psychosocial club. Two groups clinic staff (receptionists not health professionals) and clinic patients administered surveys. The first 305 surveyed by staff were randomly selected	Preliminary findings suggest that involving consumers as surveyors in satisfaction studies may produce findings that differs from those in studies with non-professional staff surveyors
Segal et al. (2002) Psychiatric Services	Primary study, level III; comparative study, USA It compared the characteristics and past service use of new enrollees of self-help agencies and community mental health agencies in the same geographical catchment Interview assessments were conducted with 673 new users at ten pairs of self-help (n=226) and community mental health agencies (n=447) serving the same geographical areas. Client characteristics were evaluated with multivariate analyses of variance and chi-squared tests	Clients of community mental health agencies had more acute symptoms, lower levels of social functioning, and more life stressors in the previous 30 days than clients of self-help agencies. The self-help agency cohort evidenced greater self-esteem, locus of control, and hope about the future. Clients of self-help agencies had received more services from facilities other than self-help or community mental health agencies in the last six months, and clients of self-help agencies who were not African American had more long-term mental health service histories Although self-help and community mental health agencies deliver primarily acute treatment-focused services, whereas self-help agencies provide services aimed at fostering socialisation, mutual support, empowerment, and autonomy

Descriptive studies

Most of the descriptive studies (e.g., Hutchison & Pedlar, 1999; Bentley, 2000) were conducted to increase understanding about users of such programmes, their demographics and their perceptions of how self-help or service-user-run programmes affected their lives. Generally speaking, respondents indicated that being involved in a service-user-run programme had a positive effect on their quality of life. High levels of satisfaction were found, and participants felt they actually ran the centres (Mowbray & Tan, 1993). Two studies focused on specific populations of interest. Petr and associates (2000) conducted an exploratory study looking at the needs, activities, structure and purposes of a consumer-run organisation for young people. A qualitative study of a peer-support programme for people with recurring mental health and substance use disorders found that benefits included developing interpersonal competence, by helping others in their recovery and giving back to others, by gaining a sense of helping people in the community by helping others grow and change and by building long-term relationships with other consumers (Salzer & Shear, 2002). Bentley (2000) undertook a preliminary evaluation of training programmes run in conjunction with a peer-run drop-in centre on a small sample ($n=10$). They attempted to look at outcomes in relation to the training, but no specific measures or scales were used to assess its effectiveness.

These selected studies were all descriptive and low in the hierarchy of evidence for determining intervention effectiveness; however, given the dearth of research in this area, they are very important in indicating the potential for service development and evaluation. They highlight several important lessons. First, successful programmes have to be run by consumers who have control of their own budget, staff and activities. Meaningful service user activities have to be integrated within the wider system. Second, prospective, longitudinal studies are required to establish if consumer-led intervention positively affects sense of empowerment, self-direction or other outcomes such as clients' service satisfaction. Segal and colleagues (1997) looked at the development of a scale that assesses clients' satisfaction with services and their involvement in treatment decisions. The Self-Help Agency Satisfaction Scale (SHASS) is a brief instrument that can be used to measure clients' satisfaction with their involvement in treatment in mental health self-help agencies, and the scale and its subscales showed high internal consistency, moderate stability and discriminant validity. Third, although there is an urgent need to assess the effectiveness of consumer-operated services, according to standard evaluation practice, parallel descriptive and process studies are also needed to document how consumer-run programmes operate, what they do and the mechanisms through which they affect consumer outcomes (Mowbray *et al.*, 2002). Fourth, there is a need for training and skill development for former service users wishing to participate in mental health service delivery. Furthermore, it is vital to tackle stigma against staff members with experience of mental illness and the lack of appropriate remuneration, which contributes to the burnout of activists and promotes over-reliance on the use of volunteers.

Comparative studies

There were two comparative studies investigating the value of having service users on a case management team. Chinman and associates (2000) looked at the outcomes of services provided by case managers who were mental health service users and case managers who were not service users. Felton *et al.* (1995) examined whether employing mental health consumers as peer specialists in an intensive case management programme could enhance outcomes for clients with serious mental illness. Both studies yielded some promising outcomes. Consumers have the potential and ability to provide mental health services as members of a case management team. Clients served by such teams with peer specialists demonstrated greater gains in several areas of quality of life, for example, in the area of self-image and outlook and social support, and in an overall reduction in the number of major life problems experienced. They also reported more frequent contacts with their case managers. Similarly, Lyons and colleagues (1996) investigated consumer service delivery in a mobile assessment programme designed to assist homeless people with severe psychiatric disorders. Staff with personal consumer experience were more likely to do street outreach, were more willing and better able to engage with mentally ill people on the street than were non-consumer staff.

Interpreting outcome data from these types of studies is not straightforward. For example, Chinman and associates (2001) described the Welcome Basket Program and reported preliminary outcome data from a pilot study to evaluate its effectiveness. It was found that at baseline the Welcome Basket Program participants were initially at greater risk for re-hospitalisation than those in standard care; however, the intervention might help reduce hospitalisation rates in this at risk population.

The remaining two studies in this review examined different aspects of service users' experiences and their implications. Polowczyk and associates (1993) compared the use of consumer interviewers and staff interviewers. Their preliminary findings suggested that, although the training received by interviewers was the same, involving service users to survey consumers in satisfaction studies might produce findings that differ from those in studies with non-professional staff surveyors. Segal and his team (2002) contrasted the characteristics and past service use of new enrollees of self-help agencies and community mental health agencies in the same region. Significant differences in psychological functioning and empowerment/attitudes were observed. They suggested that, although self-help and community mental health agencies both delivered primarily acute treatment-focused services, a critical difference was that self-help agencies appeared to provide services aimed more at fostering socialisation, mutual support, empowerment and autonomy.

Controlled studies

A randomised, controlled trial by Klein and colleagues (1998) examined a peer social support programme for high risk, dually diagnosed clients. Findings suggested that coupling peer social support with intensive case management was associated with more positive system outcomes. The peer-support structures and outcome measures used are also relevant for consumers without substance abuse. In addition, this study, although small, did use a randomisation procedure, and so it is one of the few studies to use a randomised controlled design in this area. The length of the follow-up was 6 months, and it is reasonable to assume that a longer follow-up might yield more valuable data. Paulson and associates (1999) compared the practice patterns of consumer and non-consumer providers of assertive community treatment using both quantitative and qualitative data as part of a randomised trial. The study aimed to determine whether the teams differed in the type and amount of time spent on each of tasks performed. The consumer team culture emphasised being there with the client, while the non-consumer team was more concerned with accomplishing tasks. Consumers were more flexible and relaxed in terms of schedules and not as task-oriented, although they still accomplished allocated tasks. Staff turnover and absences were higher on the consumer team, while non-consumers were more consistent in the hours they worked. Solomon and Draine (1996) examined whether a team of mental health consumers delivered intensive case management services differently from a team of non-consumer case managers. Their findings support the contention that service users can provide client-centred and service-oriented case management services using a service planning and monitoring model. However, this study did not address whether consumers could effectively also provide a clinical case management model.

Extending previous studies, Campbell (2004) conducted a multi-site randomised, controlled research trial involving 1827 participants with severe and persistent mental illness in the US. This research addressed a number of methodological limitations of previous investigations by ensuring good sample size, incorporating multiple locations covering a range of mental health facilities such as drop-in centres and educational/advocacy/mutual support programmes and applying the most stringent test of treatment effectiveness – the development and inclusion of recovery-oriented outcome measures and a fidelity test to make sure the service-led programmes did what they claimed to do. The initial findings are promising. Participants in the experimental conditions that consisted of service-user led programmes offered in addition to traditional mental health services showed greater improvement in well-being than participants in the control condition consisting of traditional mental health services only.

One Australian controlled study was found. O'Donnell and colleagues (1999) investigated the provision of client-focused services to community-based clients with schizophrenia and bipolar disorder. Clients referred for case management were randomly allocated to one of three groups: standard case management, client-focused case management or client-focused case management plus consumer advocacy. While there were no differences between the groups on quantitative measures of functioning, disability, quality of life, service satisfaction and burden of care, there were significant between-group differences on qualitative measures of satisfaction with services. The group receiving client-focused case management reported greater satisfaction with service delivery. Client-focused services were developed using an empowerment model of case management and by the addition of consumer advocates whose role was to encourage the client's self-confidence, provide role models for their recovery, enhance their communication with case managers and participate in recovery agreement meetings. The study was limited by its sample size and high attrition. This was not thought to be related to severity of illness but was more likely to be due to transience and co-morbid substance abuse in the population studied.

In contrast, Clark *et al.* (1999) compared two methods of collecting data on client satisfaction with mental health services provided by case managers and by physicians. A satisfaction survey instrument was developed with input from clients. No difference between the two groups was found in overall satisfaction with services received. Clients from both facilities reported high levels of satisfaction regardless of the interviewer, but clients reported more negative responses when interviewed by consumers.

Most of the controlled studies in this review focused on consumer participation services where the emphasis was on alternative models of case management. Consumers in these studies were working primarily within mainstream mental health services but were not necessarily employed in services where consumers were the majority in leadership roles or retained overall governance. One further study focused on using consumers as interviewers in service evaluation. The strength of these studies is that they all used random assignment to groups and a control group but sample size was often relatively small across all the groups studied. Low initial response rates and high attrition rates throughout the course of the studies emphasise the need for very large sample populations to ensure the representativeness of these types of studies. Selection criteria should also be kept broad to be meaningful.

Overall comments

When interpreting the aforementioned results, one has to be cautious about the heterogeneity of research methods utilised and of the CRSs (Goldstrom *et al.*, 2006). For example, sometimes the CRSs operated as adjuncts to traditional mental health services, whereas others were stand-alone programmes. The most striking feature of CRSs profiled here is, that on the whole, it led to improved levels of satisfaction among the users. Another important finding is that consumer-run or consumer-led services have not been shown to have any harmful effects on service users.

Other general benefits of consumers-run services included improvements in:

■ Well-being and quality of life.
■ Self-image and outlook about life.
■ Social support.
■ Developing the confidence and competence to help others and build long-term relationships.
■ General psychological functioning.
■ Perceived empowerment and autonomy.
■ An overall reduction in the number of major life problems.

There were also benefits to the services themselves such as adoption of a more client-centred practice and services became more accessible, user-friendly and more active in reaching out to consumers. Another benefit is that CRSs are useful in reaching individuals who do not use or willingly engage with traditional mental health services.

This review used a structured approach to review the literature and the scope was confined to an examination of the effectiveness of the service or programme. Although this chapter does not consider the acceptability, or any ethical, economic or legal considerations associated with CRSs or programmes, these are important issues worthy of further study. The majority of the reviewed articles were written by professionals with or without input from consumers, which might have influenced how the study was designed and the outcomes measured. In turn, the results reported might not fully reflect or capture consumers' experience in consumer-run or consumer-operated services. Qualitative studies were not included as they are not designed to quantify the effectiveness of services. However, qualitative research is useful in providing a rich description of how CRSs are delivered, the unique experience and perceptions of service providers and consumers, and the specific context of individual programmes. Although a number of descriptive studies were included, the range of programmes examined for this level of evidence should be considered a cross-section of those available, as retrieval for these types of studies was selective rather than exhaustive. There are other informative, descriptive studies that contribute to the emerging research base for peer-run support programmes, but they have not been summarised in this review.

Occupational therapists' contribution to enhance consumers-run mental health services

Swarbrick and Pratt (2006) summarise the potential roles and opportunities for occupational therapists to collaborate with consumer-run services as follows:

■ Work with other mental health professionals to advocate for funding for developing consumer-run services where there are none in the local area.
■ Be aware of the range of consumer-run services available in the local community.
■ Refer clients to consumer-run agencies and help establish more formalised referral procedures.
■ Promote the philosophies and use of consumer-run services among individuals in recovery from mental illness, families and with professionals and colleagues.
■ Contribute to consumer-run services research, for example, by examining outcomes.

Tse (2006) presented a paper at The New Zealand Association of Occupational Therapists Conference when there was discussion about the key challenges for establishing consumer-run services and the contribution of occupational therapists to make it happen. This section captures the key points from the dialogues between the presenter and the conference delegates.

Address challenges and minimise barriers

Occupational therapists can support colleagues working in consumer-run services to address the following challenges and barriers.

Stigma and discrimination

Stigma and discrimination against consumers who work in mental health settings comes from two sources. Firstly, some mental health professionals may have difficulty accepting the idea of consumers working with them as their colleagues. Secondly, within the service user community, there may be a paradox whereby some consumers may think they need to have serious mental health problems before they are recognised as able to provide input or leadership to a consumer-run programme. Alternatively, if the individuals are mentally well and capable of work, they may no longer be regarded as 'one of us'. This paradox places pressure on consumers in addition to the practicalities of ensuring the smooth running of a consumer-run programme.

Marginalisation

Sometimes consumers working in mental health are marginalised by the system they are employed by. This leads to limited consumer participation in the development of policies and services and restricts opportunity to effect meaningful changes in the health care system. For example, consumer consultants can be seen as a 'later addition to an already established legislative and policy framework' (Middleton *et al.*, 2004, p. 510). CRSs may be seen as second-class, low-status services and, consequently, may be poorly funded and resourced.

Accountability

Accountability becomes an issue as CRSs are funded by the mental health system and individual workers are responsible to employers. CRSs are not directly accountable to service users as a collective group, creating tension between individual staff working in CRSs and the consumers they represent or work for.

Complexities of the mental health system

'The mental health system with its legislative basis, and bureaucratic and hierarchical organisation, is difficult to understand' (Middleton *et al.*, 2004, p. 510). Individuals working in CRSs may not have had the opportunity of education within a specific health discipline that provides an understanding of this complex and changing mental health system.

Domination of biomedical model

The biomedical model is rooted in patriarchal power structures that assume that experts know what is best for patients. Patients are considered as passive recipients of services rather than individuals who actively construct the meaning of their experiences. In turn, some mental health professionals are reluctant or unwilling to consider consumers' views or to work collaboratively with them. There are many situations in health care where medical knowledge and skills are invaluable and life-saving; however, excessive professional domination often undermines what CRSs can offer to individuals in recovery.

Becoming unwell

Another dilemma faced by individuals working in CRSs is that the experience of mental health problems, which qualify the person to work in such services in the first place, may interfere with the performance of their roles. This has a number of implications. Consumers can become unwell or unable to continue with their role in the service, but it may be unclear how much of their illness is due to mental health problems or difficulties encountered in their role. When unwell, consumers may be unclear as to whom to go to for support or they may be in a position of sole responsibility with no one to delegate tasks to. They may feel disconnected and isolated in their role. Lastly, on returning to work after an acute episode of illness, the acceptance by their own colleagues, both consumers and non-consumers, and also the consumer community is of paramount importance.

Burnout

Mental health workers may experience exhaustion, diminished interest or increased level of cynicism in the work context. People working in CRSs are no exception to this experience and perhaps they may be more prone to burnout and compassion fatigue than their counterparts because they not only deal with the stress associated with everyday work and their personal health problems but also potential workplace discrimination.

Find the right people

For a CRS to flourish it is important to attract people with the right mix of skills, experience and training.

Most of these issues do not stem from the choice to provide a consumer-run service itself. To address them effectively, a strategic approach is needed to identify the problems and implement an action and evaluation plan. Consumers, managers, planners, providers and clinicians need to work together at all levels to make CRSs a reality. Some workplace culture or practices have to be questioned, and those currently responsible for services have to accept that power and resources must be shared to make CRSs work.

Adopt a collaborative approach and contribute to 'Service Green' environment

Middleton and his colleagues (2004) conducted in-depth, semi-structured interviews with ten consumer consultants to explore areas of influence, areas of difficulty and suggestions for improvement. Based on the data, the researchers developed

Table 12.4 Characteristics of 'Green Services', 'Apathetic Services' and 'Red Services' representing different levels of support to consumers-run services (CRS).

Green Services: collaborative and enabling, characterised by	Apathetic Services: no support and no obstruction, characterised by	Red Services: rigid and unresponsive, characterised by
• Members from CRS attend management committee	• Management and clinical team is either neutral or apathetic to CRS	• Members from CRS are not welcome to attend management committee
• CRS controls and is accountable for their own budget	• Management and clinical team accepts CRS but does little to promote or actively support the services	• If attend, CRS items are discussed last minute or frequently deferred
• Employees of CRS are on reasonable pay and work full time whenever possible	• Staff are not obstructive to CRS	• CRS has no control of their own budget
• CRS feels supported by management and employees choose their own regular supervision (paid by the CRS budget)	• Conduct consultations and feedback from service users but do nothing to improve the services in the light of comments	• Employees of CRS are not on reasonable pay and offered part-time position only due to 'budget constraint'
• Staff value CRS		• CSR feels unsupported by management; supervision is either imposed rigidly (e.g. who is the supervisor) or virtually non-existent
• CRS actively seeks feedback from service users and present them in management committee		• Staff oppose CRS
• Management and clinical teams incorporate broader approaches to mental illness		• CRS is discouraged to seek feedback from service users or present them in management committee
• Management and clinical teams are favourable to the multi-disciplinary team		• Management and clinical teams adopt paternalistic attitudes towards consumers or CRS if exist
• CRS can provide meaningful inputs in relation to service users treatment issue (if applicable)		• Domination of medical model in the multi-disciplinary team
		• CRS is discouraged to provide inputs in relation to service users treatment issue

Source: Middleton *et al.* (2004, p. 516).

the three service typologies: Service Green, which has characteristics favourable to consumer participation; Apathetic Service, where staff are neutral about consumer participation and Service Red, with less favourable characteristics. Table 12.4 highlights the key characteristics of each type that may be used to assess services.

Although, no existing services would correspond exactly with this three-fold typology, this framework can help planners and providers to clarify the challenges and actions are required to facilitate a favourable environment for development of CRSs in mental health.

Summary

This review of the effectiveness of consumer-run mental health services found a mixed record of research. Descriptive studies support the feasibility of these types of services but only a limited number of studies focus on outcomes for people who receive services from consumers. They report positive outcomes for their clients with no harmful effects. A very good case for their inclusion in the array of services offered within the mental health can be made based on recent findings from controlled studies, particularly that of Campbell (2004).

Consumers should determine the style of consumer-run services to be developed and should already have meaningful input into existing service structures. The reality may be different. Occupational therapists and others can be advocates for the continued support of existing consumer providers and can assist in the development of new services through the provision of material resources, support and possibly staff. Ultimately, as Mowbray and Tan (1993) suggest, it is the mental health consumers themselves who will create the services and make them work.

Consumer-run mental health services promote consumers offering peer support to other consumers. This is an area that is attracting international attention, but maintaining its non-professional vantage point may be crucial in helping people with mental health problems rebuild their sense of identity and community (Mead & MacNeill, 2004). The development of CRSs and the practice of peer support create a platform from which people with mental health problems can share their unique perspectives. Consumers are aware that they must not change the nature of intentional peer support simply because of pressure to legitimise or justify CRSs to traditional providers (Mead, 2006). The history of peer support is of a culture that emerged as a response to doing things differently (Campbell, 2005) so that the CRSs and peer-support programmes of the future need not look or feel like clones of current services. The challenge for everyone who works in mental health services is not to fear a shift from how services incorporate consumer knowledge and participation at present but to remain open to the different ways in which this might happen in the future.

Questioning your Practice

1. What are the general findings about the effectiveness of consumer-run services?
2. How are consumer-run services contributing to favourable rehabilitation outcomes for individuals in recovery from mental health problems?
3. How can occupational therapists support the development and delivery of consumer-run services?

References

Bentley KJ (2000) Empowering Our Own: peer leadership training for a drop-in center. *Psychiatric Rehabilitation Journal, 24(2)*, 174–178.

Campbell J (2004) *Consumer-Operated Services Programs (CoSP) Multsite Research Initiative: Overview and Preliminary Findings.* St Louis, MO: Missouri Institute of Mental Health, University of Missouri School of Medicine. Retrieved 16 July 2007 http://www.cstprogram.org/consumer%20.p/index.html (retrieved July 16, 2007).

Campbell J (2005) The historical and philosophical development of peer-run support programs. In: S Clay, S. Bonnie, P Corrigan, R Ralph (eds) *On Our Own, Together: Peer Programs for People with Mental Illness.* Nashville, TN: Vanderbilt University Press, pp. 17–64.

Chamberlin J, Rogers ES, Ellison ML (1996) Self-help programs: A description of their characteristics and their members. *Psychiatric Rehabilitation Journal, 19(3)*, 33–42.

Chen H (1990) *Theory-Driven Evaluations.* Newbury Park, CA: Sage.

Chinman MJ, Rosenheck R, Lam JA, Davidson L (2000) Comparing consumer and nonconsumer provided case management services for homeless persons with serious mental illness. *Journal of Nervous and Mental Disease, 188(7)*, 446–453.

Chinman MJ, Weingarten R, Stayner D, Davidson L (2001) Chronicity reconsidered: improving person-environment fit through a consumer-run service. *Community Mental Health Journal, 37(3)*, 215–229.

Clark CC, Scott EA, Boydell KM, Goering P (1999) Effects of client interviewers on client-reported satisfaction with mental health services. *Psychiatric Services, 50(7)*, 961–963.

Clay S (ed.) (2005) *On Our Own Together: Peer Programs for People with Mental Illness.* Nashville, TN: Vanderbilt University Press.

Cook JA, Jonikas JA, Razzano L (1995) A randomized evaluation of consumer versus nonconsumer training of state mental health service providers. *Community Mental Health Journal, 31(3)*, 229–238.

Corr S, Neill G, Turner A (2005) Comparing an occupational therapy definition and consumer's experiences: a Q methodology study. *British Journal of Occupational Therapy, 68(8)*, 338–346.

Davidson L, Chinman M, Kloos B, Weingarten R, Stayner D, Tebes JK (1999) Peer support among individuals with severe mental illness: A review of the evidence. *Clinical Psychology-Science and Practice, 6(2)*, 165–187.

Department of Health and Community Services (1996) *Victorian Mental Health Service Working with Consumers. Guidelines for Consumer Participation in Mental HealthServices,* Melbourne, Australia: Psychiatric Service Division, Government of Victoria.

Felton CJ, Stastny P, Shern DL, Blanch A, Donahve SA, Knight E, Brown C (1995) Consumers as peer specialists on intensive case management teams: impact on client outcomes. *Psychiatric Services, 46(10),* 1037–1044.

Fossey EM, Harvey CA (2001) A conceptual review of functioning: implications for the development of consumer outcome measures. *Australian and New Zealand Journal of Psychiatry,* 35(1), 91–98.

Goldstrom ID, Campbell J, Rogers JA, Lambert DB, Blacklow B, Henderson MJ, Manderscheid RW (2006) National estimates for mental health mutual support groups, self-help organizations, and consumer-operated services. *Administration and Policy in Mental Health and Mental Health Services Research, 33(1),* 92–103.

Honey A (1999) Empowerment versus power: consumer participation in mental health services. *Occupational Therapy International, 6(4),* 257–276.

Hutchison P, Pedlar A (1999) Independent living centres: an innovation with mental health implications? *Canadian Journal of Community Mental Health, 18(2),* 21–32.

Klein AR, Cnaan RA, Whitecraft J (1998) Significance of peer social support with dually diagnosed clients: findings from a pilot study. *Research on Social Work Practice, 8(5),* 529–551.

Lyons JS, Cook JA, Ruth AR, Karver M, Slagg NB (1996) Service delivery using consumer staff in a mobile crisis assessment program. *Community Mental Health Journal, 32,* 33–40.

MacNeil C, Abbott K (2000) *An Evaluation of the Peer Specialist Initiative.* Albany, NY: New York State Office of Mental Health, Bureau of Recipient Affairs.

Mead S (2006) *Intentional peer support: an alternative approach. Manual for Balance NZ – Bipolar and Depression Network.* Peer Support Training Days (21–24 September 2006) Wanganui, New Zealand.

Mead S, MacNeill C (2004) *Peer Support: What Makes it Unique?* Unpublished article.

Meehan T, Bergen H, Coveney C, *et al.* (2002) Development and evaluation of a training program in peer support for former consumers. *International Journal of Mental Health Nursing, 11(1),* 34–39.

Middleton P, Stanton P, Renouf N (2004) Consumer Consultants in mental health services: address the challenges. *Journal of Mental Health, 13(5),* 507–518.

Mowbray CT, Tan C (1993) Consumer-operated drop-in centers: evaluation of operations and impact. *Journal of Mental Health Administration, 20(1),* 8–19.

Mowbray CT, Holter MC, Stark L, Pfeffer C, Bybee D (2005) A Fidelity rating Instrument for Consumer-run Drop-in Centers (FRI-CRDI). *Research on Social Work Practice, 15(4),* 278–290.

Mowbray CT, Robinson EA, Holter MC (2002) Consumer drop-in centers: operations, services, and consumer involvement. *Health & Social Work, 27(4),* 248–261.

Mueser K, Glynn S, Corrigan P, Baber W (1996) A survey of preferred terms for users of mental health services. *Psychiatric Services, 47(7),* 760–761.

National Health and Medical Research Council (2000) *How To Use the Evidence: Assessment and Application of Scientific Evidence.* Canberra, Australia: NHMRC.

O'Donnell M, Parker G, Proberts M, Matthews R (1999) A study of client-focused case management and consumer advocacy: the Community and Consumer Service Project. *Australian & New Zealand Journal of Psychiatry, 33(5),* 684–693.

Oakley Browne MA, Wells JE, Scott KM (eds) (2006) *Te Rau Hinengaro: The New Zealand Mental Health Survey.* Wellington, New Zealand: Ministry of Health.

Paulson R, Henrickx H, Demmler J, Clarke G, Cutler D, Birecree E (1999) Comparing practice patterns of consumer and non-consumer mental health service providers. *Community Mental Health Journal, 35(3),* 251–269.

Petr CG, Holtquist S, Martin JS (2000) Consumer-run organizations for youth. *Psychiatric Rehabilitation Journal, 24(2)*, 142–148.

Polowczyk D, Brutus M, Orvieto A, Vidul J, Cipriani D (1993) Comparison of patient and staff surveys of consumer satisfaction. *Hospital & Community Psychiatry, 44(6)*, 589–591.

Salzer MS, Shear SL (2002) Identifying consumer-provider benefits in evaluations of consumer-delivered services. *Psychiatric Rehabilitation Journal, 25(3)*, 281–288.

Segal SP, Silverman C (2002) Determinants of client outcomes in self-help agencies. *Psychiatric Services, 53(3)*, 304–309.

Segal SP, Redman D, Silverman C (2000) Measuring clients' satisfaction with self-help agencies. *Psychiatric Services, 51(9)*, 1148–1152.

Segal SP, Silverman C, Temkin T (1997) Program environments of self-help agencies for persons with mental disabilities. *Journal of Mental Health Administration, 24(4)*, 456–464.

Simpson EL, House AO (2002) Involving users in the delivery and evaluation of mental health services: systematic review. *British Medical Journal, 325(2)*, 1265.

Simpson EL, House AO (2003) User and carer involvement in mental health services: from rhetoric to science. *British Journal of Psychiatry, 183(2)*, 89–91.

Solomon P, Draine J (1996) Service delivery differences between consumer and nonconsumer case managers in mental health. *Research on Social Work Practice, 6(2)*, 193–207.

Sumsion T (1999) *Client-Centred Practice in Occupational Therapy*. Philadelphia: Elsevier Health Sciences.

Swarbrick P, Pratt C (2006) Consumer-operated self-help services: roles and opportunities for occupational therapists and occupational therapy assistants. *OT Practice, 11(5)*, CE1–8.

Tobin M, Chen L, Leathley C (2002) Consumer participation in mental health services: who wants it and why? *Australian Health Review, 25(3)*, 91–100.

Torrey WC, Mead S, Ross G (1998) Addressing the social needs of mental health consumers when day treatment programs convert to supported employment: can consumer-run services play a role? *Psychiatric Rehabilitation Journal, 22(1)*, 73–75.

Tse S (2006) Therapeutic use of self: Consumer-run mental health services: does it work or is it just PC (politically correct)? Paper presented at the New Zealand Association of Occupational Therapists Conference, Te Papa, Wellington, New Zealand, 2 September 2006.

13 Twists and turns
The development of a clinical–academic career pathway

Edward A.S. Duncan

Personal narrative

My entry into occupational therapy was completely serendipitous. I had left school at 17 years of age, having failed to achieve anything of academic significance. After 3 years of mundane administrative positions, in the civil service and with a stockbroker, I was searching for a professional direction in my life. I had held a desire to work in the health care field from an early age, but was really at a loss to know in what capacity. One evening, whilst at a friend's house party, I met a friendly and attractive girl. Looking for an excuse to continue speaking to her I asked her what she was studying; occupational therapy, she replied. What is that, I asked. By the time the party had finished I realised that, whilst the girl and I had no future, I had discovered my professional destiny!

But I was faced with a challenge. Academically I came nowhere near the required entrance qualifications. I began to search for opportunities, and luck was on my side. An access course designed to support people in just my position had recently been designed and was looking for applicants. To gain a place one had to be accepted by both the College of Further Education and the Occupational Therapy Department at Queen Margaret College (QMC), Edinburgh. The course had been set up with the support of Averil Stewart, then the Head of the Occupational Therapy Department at QMC and later the UK's first professor of occupational therapy. A series of applications and interviews followed. Much to my surprise and delight I was awarded a place, and I embarked on an opportunity I never imagined would come my way, undertaking a degree in a higher education. Perhaps because of this relatively late academic start – I was 21 years of age when I commenced my degree and my new found potential for learning – I entered my undergraduate education with great enthusiasm.

I am naturally inquisitive. From my earliest student days on the occupational therapy course I clearly understood that I wanted to undertake a PhD and pursue a clinical–academic/research career. This was slightly unusual, although it did not feel so at the time, as there was not really such a thing as a clinical–academic/research career pathway. Yet I was aware of burning questions that could only be answered through research and I was determined to participate in answering them. Equally apparent from very early on was my interest in mental health. This interest was fostered both through the inspiring lectures of Dr Sheena Blair, now Head of Department of Occupational Therapy at Glasgow Caledonian University, who held the main responsibility for lecturing on mental health topics, and through a range of fascinating practice placements. Sheena holds a particular interest in psychodynamic approaches (Blair & Daniel, 2006), and I remember leaving her lectures and tutorials with my head bursting with thoughts and reflections on what we had learnt and discussed. Undoubtedly, her imparting of psychodynamic approaches was a strong foundation for my early understanding of mental health theory and interpersonal dynamics, and it provided knowledge and understanding that have held me in good stead throughout my career to date.

I left college after 4 years, the traditional length of an honours degree in Scotland, determined to get a job as an occupational therapist in mental health. I did not care too much in what field it was, although I was particularly interested in working in child and adolescent psychiatry, as I had previously completed a practice placement with Gita Ingram (Ingram, 2003), which I had found particularly fascinating. About the only mental health area of practice I held no desire to work in was forensic psychiatry. A fellow student had recently undertaken her elective placement at Broadmoor Hospital in the newly opened forensic occupational therapy department. I clearly remember telling her that that was one area I held absolutely no desire to work in; as time was to tell I was obviously as poor an assessor of my future professional interests as I had previously been of my academic ability!

Early clinical positions

My formative clinical experiences as a qualified occupational therapist were in two community mental health teams (CMHT) in Glasgow. The first team was based in Rutherglen, an historic Royal Burgh on the outskirts of the city, and the second team was in the Gorbals, an infamous inner city area, which was just beginning to undergo significant regeneration. Both teams included catchment areas of significant social deprivation. As is so typical of occupational therapists working in community mental health teams (Harries & Gilhooly, 2003a), my caseload was a mixture of generic and occupational therapy specific cases. Entering the reality of peoples' lives in these areas was an eye opener for me. Whilst I thoroughly enjoyed my work, I often felt as if I was helping people deal with functional challenges that despite my best efforts were unlikely to significantly ease. So many issues, on top of whatever mental illness they had, appeared largely out of my control. Poverty, familial drug and alcohol difficulties, poor housing and unemployment, amongst a range of other issues, all appeared to be stacked against many of the clients I worked with. Issues such as occupational alienation, occupational injustice or occupational deprivation had yet to be clearly articulated in the occupational science literature. However, it dawned on me that if I truly wanted to make a difference to these peoples' mental health, I should have become a town planner or a politician. And yet the value of the small gains that people made in their lives through engaging in occupational therapy were also apparent. Both health promotion and rehabilitation are required to support people lives. Occupational therapists can and do become involved in a range of activities that support health promotion. However, whilst such activities are laudable and undeniably necessary, if occupational therapists concentrated on these issues, they would dilute their expertise. Occupational therapy, I concluded, should focus on helping people who are occupationally dysfunctional and should not be distracted in this task by the broader aim of promoting a healthy society; other professionals have greater expertise in this area.

One thing was clear though: the average client who was referred to the CMHTs I worked in had little time for a psychodynamic perspective of their difficulties. I had to acknowledge that psychodynamic theory, though still useful in helping me understand a variety of situations and dynamics, was of little practical use in the clinical situations in which I worked as a newly qualified occupational therapist. For example, there was a lady in a thirteenth floor flat who had an on-going psychotic illness, whose self-care and activities of daily living had deteriorated significantly and who had not left her flat in weeks. The pile of rotting foodstuffs piled on the floor, up to her window, could literally be seen to be crawling. Or alternatively, there was the 19-year-old mother who, after leaving her violent partner, was in a hostel looking after her three young children and was experiencing anxiety and depression and was on the verge of recommencing a damaging drug habit. What was required in these situations was a practical and evidence-based theoretical approach that I could actively use with such individuals. Unsurprisingly, I found myself strongly attracted by cognitive-behavioural therapy (CBT), not least because of its compelling evidence base, practical focus and resonance with occupational therapy. I began to incorporate its principles in my practice. I was not as concerned as others about the potential for role blurring throughout the use of shared frames of reference. Indeed, I saw such developments as a natural consequence for some occupational therapists (Duncan, 1999). My interest in CBT has continued, but my understanding of its place and role in occupational therapy has significantly developed (Duncan 2003a, 2006a). It was my interest in pursuing a postgraduate diploma in cognitive-behavioural psychotherapy at the University of Dundee that ultimately led to my next, and unexpected, clinical career move – from community to forensic mental health.

Developing research skills

Having spent 2 years working in adult community mental health teams in Glasgow, I went to work at The State Hospital, Carstairs. 'The State Hospital provides treatment and care in conditions of special security for individuals with mental disorder who, because of their dangerous, violent or criminal propensities, cannot be cared for in any other setting' (The State Hospitals Board for Scotland, 2002, p. 3). It is located in rural Scotland, about one hour drive from both Glasgow and Edinburgh.

There were many attractions that enticed me to work there, despite my previous reservations about forensic care. The hospital was in the throes of increasing its therapeutic focus, and as part of that process was re-establishing its occupational therapy department after several fallow years, during which no occupational therapists had worked in the hospital. Both the hospital management and the newly appointed head occupational therapist were determined to make the new occupational therapy department a success. As part of this process, several premises were set. The new department was to make a positive contribution to patient care, to embrace the use of theory in practice and to encourage and support research. As offending behaviour rehabilitation is strongly influenced by CBT, there was also the opportunity to complete the postgraduate training I had been so eager to do.

One of the strengths of the newly established occupational therapy department at The State Hospital was the appointment of a critical mass of therapists who were all committed to the agenda of incorporating theory into practice and using and developing research as a core component of practice. The development of the department is described in greater depth elsewhere (Urquhart, 2003). In this chapter I wish to focus on its development of research in practice. Recognising the need for academic support, the department employed Dr Maggie Nicol, now professor and head of the department at Queen Margaret University College, Edinburgh, to act as a research supervisor. Maggie attended the department most months for almost 5 years. Her remit was broadly to assist staff to develop their own research projects. These spanned a range of activities from assisting support staff to develop skills in critical appraisal of journal papers to becoming my PhD supervisor. Maggie's collaboration with the department supported the staff to become involved in a range of research activities including conference presentations and small research projects.

Having completed my postgraduate diploma in cognitive-behavioural psychotherapy, my academic enthusiasm was unabated and I decided to embark on a part-time PhD. I was fortunate as I was working in a department that valued research, and therefore, to a certain extent, my interest in pursuing a PhD was understood. The department supported me by giving me one day a week to focus on my research, and I applied for and was successful in gaining my first research grant to cover my fees and training expenses. At the outset of my doctoral studies, I imagined that on completion of my PhD I would probably become an occupational therapy lecturer. This is not in itself surprising as the vast majority of role models I had of occupational therapists with PhDs were lecturers.

My original intention was to study, the efficacy of cognitive-behavioural psychotherapy in enhancing the level of social competency in a population of sexual offenders against children, who had a concurrent mental illness. This topic was chosen as it was related to my previous CBT studies, was relevant to the clinical context in which I worked and was fundable. Holloway and Walker (2000), suggest that the rationale for selecting a research topic should be based on factors such as:

■ A problem or issue identified in practice.
■ A professional issue which has intrigued the researcher.

- Issues that emerge from the literature.
- Issues that have emerged from previous academic study.
- Interest stimulated by personal knowledge or experience.

Whilst I was able to tick all these boxes in relation to my planned study, after 2 years of work it became apparent that this topic was neither practically or politically feasible.

Previous outcome studies had been carried out within the hospital (Donnelly & Guy, 1998; Donnelly & Scott, 1999; Donnelly *et al.*, 2001). However, these studies examined interventions that patients had been referred to as part of their routine care, and consequently consent to participate was high, with few patients refusing to participate. My proposed randomised control study was to be the first outcome study within the hospital that had not occurred as part of ongoing care and treatment and as such there was no intrinsic gain for patients from participation. Whilst recruitment to the study was expected to be a challenging issue, there were no other studies available within the institution from which to predict a baseline recruitment rate. The lower-than-expected recruitment rate to the study significantly affected the practical feasibility of this strand of the thesis.

Another issue, which I had not considered at the outset, was the study's political feasibility. Delamont *et al.* (1997) considered 'political feasibility' to include factors that are sensitive to the institution or professional bodies concerned. At the commencement of the research, the proposed sample population of sexual offenders were not a priority intervention group within the hospital. However, The Mental Welfare Commission (2000) reported on the care a discharged patient received, whilst in The State Hospital. This report resulted in significant changes within the hospital. Amongst these was the development of several new group interventions for specific patient populations, including sexual offenders. This population therefore moved from being a known, but underevaluated patient population, to a high-profile population, which currently receives the longest group intervention within the hospital.[1] Delamont *et al.* (1997) stated that, under such circumstances, this type of research is only feasible if the appropriate 'gatekeepers' specifically request it. As this was not the case, several organisational difficulties were encountered. Consequently, my PhD studies were broadened and changed direction to focus on group interventions with mentally disordered offenders. Inevitably this was a frustrating experience, yet it also taught me several valuable research lessons. Not least of which is the necessity to have a dogged determination to conduct research and an ability to overcome hurdles and seek solutions rather than being disheartened by the setbacks that will inevitable occur. Another resolution from that time was to get the most output for any work that I carry out, and thankfully not all of my work on sexual offending went to waste (Duncan, 2003b).

A key component of developing as a clinical–academic is to publish your work. This can be a daunting experience at first. To develop this skill, I explored

---

[1] 'CORE 2000' is a group intervention for sexual offenders. This group is used within The Prison Service and has been adapted for use within The State Hospital since 2001.

opportunities to publish my research and other activities. As part of the research focus of our department I became increasingly interested and involved in examining ways to deliver evidence-based practice. In particular, I became involved in two clinical effectiveness strategies that supported evidence-based practice, namely, clinical guideline implementation and integrated care pathways. Both of these strategies were ongoing hospital developments and assisted the occupational therapy department to enable the best evidence to be used and for evidence-based practice to be monitored. I was fortunate in being able to collaborate with a range of multi-disciplinary colleagues and publish our work in this area (Duncan *et al.*, 2000; Duncan & Moody, 2003). I was also concerned that the forensic environment and client group may require a different set of research priorities to those that had previously been determined within the professions (e.g. Fowler Davis & Bannigan, 2000; Fowler Davis and Hyde, 2002). This interest in forensic research priorities led to a brief research project and the publication of a specific set of research priorities for forensic occupational therapy (Duncan *et al.*, 2003). Further collaborations with other colleagues resulted in two other publications: a survey (Bannigan and Duncan, 2001) and a clinical evaluation (Donnelly *et al.*, 2001). I was also fortunate to be able to publish some of my PhD before I submitted my thesis (Duncan *et al.*, 2004b).

Whilst my studies were perhaps the most demanding, I was certainly not alone in developing a clinical–academic career and the department's collaboration with a senior occupational therapy lecturer had proven most fruitful. Continuing evidence of the research capacity that such a collaboration can build can be seen in the flourishing Forensic Occupational Therapy Conference, which is now a core component of the business of the College of Occupational Therapists Specialist Section in Mental Health, but originated from the occupational therapy department at The State Hospital, and the fact that such research collaborations have since been replicated and continue elsewhere (Urquhart, 2003).

Despite the strengths of this clinical–academic collaboration, there were some challenges. The department's research outcomes tended to develop in an *ad hoc* fashion and according to clinicians' personal interests. Although there was management endorsement for research, it tended to be perceived by therapists as an added extra to clinical work and consequentially had not become fully integrated within the service (Duncan *et al.*, 2004). This appeared to frustrate some staff and lessened their motivation to actively participate in research. Owing to her recent promotion, Maggie Nicol, the original academic link, was unable to continue to provide the service she had. Serendipitously, Dr Kirsty Forysth, co-director of UK Centre for Outcomes Research and Education (UKCORE), had recently returned to Scotland, and the department approached UKCORE for support to deliver and generate evidence-based services in a strategically planned way.

UK CORE is conceptualised as an organisational structure to bridge academic departments and occupational therapy practice settings. It differs significantly from the original clinical–academic partnership the hospital had developed, as the focus of UKCORE was on the department and not the individual. Key aspects of this new collaboration included integrating evidence-based practice in to the everyday work of clinicians' lives, supporting them to deliver and develop evidence for practice, creating a research strategy and developing new supervisory and leadership structures (Forsyth *et al.*, 2005a). Another key component was the development of a new position within the department, head research practitioner, with a remit to support the delivery of the department's developed research strategy and deliver expert evidence-based clinical practice. The post had dedicated time for this purpose and was directly supported by UKCORE staff (Forsyth *et al.*, 2005a). I was fortunate to be asked to carry out this task, and was happy to do so as it brought together my clinical and academic interests. Research outputs continued from the department, but new opportunities also arose to participate in international research collaborations. For example, the department participated in the data collection for the reliability study of the newly published Model of Human Occupation Screening Tool (MOHOST) (Forsyth *et al.*, *paper submitted for publication*) and also collaborated in developing a forensic specific version of the Occupational Circumstances Analysis and Rating Scale (OCAIRS) (Forsyth *et al.*, 2005b). Whilst these benefits were substantial for the department and focused their research activities in a way that was arguably more useful to the patient population, it is also true that some staff missed the individual flexibility that was vital in the original academic collaboration.

By this point, I was coming towards the end of my PhD. Time had passed and new opportunities were developing for clinicians interested in developing clinical–academic career pathways. A new breed of clinician had been proposed, the consultant occupational therapist, although there were still few in existence. This position was designed to stem the flow of good clinicians from entering management and education and to develop a new leadership capacity within the allied health professions, including research leadership. I pondered career options for several months. Another new opportunity in Scotland then occurred, one that I had never considered as sufficient funding had previously been unavailable – a postdoctoral research fellowship in a centre of research excellence.

Postdoctoral research

From an initially dismissing opinion of working in forensic mental health; to plans of working in the area for a few years, I ultimately spent 9 years at The State Hospital. In itself, that is testament to how valuable and positive I found the experience. But it was clear to me that my future plans lay in developing a clinical–academic career in adult mental health, and limiting my research options to the forensic setting would be too restrictive. The opportunity to undertake a postdoctoral research fellowship seemed too good an opportunity to miss. It is fair to say that my interest in making this career move was not understood by everyone. Having recently gained my PhD, some people felt that enough had been achieved academically; why would one want to do more? Whilst historically gaining a PhD was seen as the culminating episode of a person's research career, I felt I was just getting started. My PhD was a credential – the first rung on the ladder and the future lay in developing a robust clinical–academic research career.

The Nursing Midwifery and Allied Health Professions Research Training Scheme, which organised the postdoctoral research fellowship, was funded by a consortium of funding bodies, including NHS Education for Scotland, Scottish Executive Health Department and the Health Foundation. Its inception followed the publication of the first national allied health professions research strategy for Scotland (Scottish Executive, 2004). The training scheme itself was a consortium of various universities, research units and the NHS. Potential fellows were required to develop a research proposal and training plan with one of the training consortium's departments or units and present this as part of their application process. The most appropriate research unit for my interests was the chief scientist's Nursing Midwifery and Allied Health Professions Research Unit (NMAHP RU), a national research unit funded by the chief scientist office, a branch of the Scottish Executive Health Department. I linked myself to the unit's decision-making programme at the University of Stirling and was fortunate to gain the first postdoctoral fellowship awarded by this scheme. Consequentially I was seconded from the hospital to the unit for 2 years.

Moving from conducting research as a clinician in a hospital to being a full-time researcher in a dedicated research unit was not difficult, but the change in working culture was nevertheless remarkable. From a myriad of differences that could be highlighted, two stand out: the benefit of a multi-disciplinary research team and the change in perspective of research. I will briefly discuss each in turn. Having spent recent years based within an occupational therapy department, it was a novelty to be based in a multi-disciplinary environment once again. The decision-making programme has always had a strong midwifery component and my new colleagues had clinical backgrounds in nursing and midwifery. I found this skill and knowledge mix refreshing and stimulating. Whilst our clinical interests could not be more different, we faced similar research challenges – designing appropriate studies to answer clinically relevant questions, grant writing gaining ethical and management approval for studies, conducting effective studies, analysing data and disseminating findings. The unit also has good links with a number of other academics and research groups, and regular research discussions and project developments occur in collaboration with staff bringing expertise in philosophy, decision making, psychology, statistics and applied mathematics, amongst other areas. The importance of creating multi-disciplinary links in research has recently been endorsed by the Scottish Executive (2006). From my perspective, I would now say that I could not comprehend forming a research team that consisted purely of occupational therapists.

The second key difference was a shift in perspective surrounding research activity. Whilst smaller developmental research studies are part of the work conducted by the unit, the focus is on larger quantitative studies that are designed to answer clinically relevant questions. This was and remains a steep learning curve. As a consequence of both these factors, my research ideas have developed and benefited considerably from the expertise and vision that comes with a being a part of a national research unit.

During my fellowship I was awarded a research grant to study occupational therapists' clinical judgement and decision making in adult community mental health teams. Occupational therapists routinely make decisions about their interventions with clients. However, clinicians' decisions in situations of uncertainty, such as mental health care, are known to be influenced by a range of factors (Freemantle, 1996; Grove & Meehl, 1996), such as their attitudes to structured theories and their use of standardised assessments. Consequently, therapists are inconsistent in making decisions in practice. There is therefore a need to explore ways in which a greater agreement between therapists' decisions is achieved. A range of conceptual models of practice have been developed to support occupational therapists' decision making in practice (Duncan, 2006c). These models developed out of a desire to explain why a client is experiencing a particular problem, what a potential solution could be and why a particular intervention works. Several theorists have also developed associated standardised assessments. One such assessment is the OCAIRS. Theoretically, assessments such as the OCAIRS should increase agreement amongst therapists in practice. However, this hypothesis was untested. This study aimed to ascertain whether the use of a standardised screening tool increases clinicians' consistency and agreement in their prioritisation of clients' problems requiring occupational therapy intervention within adult community mental health teams. Participants were occupational therapists working in adult community mental health teams. They were recruited throughout the UK, using occupational therapy NHS managerial structures and the membership list of the then Association of Occupational Therapists in Mental Health, now the College of Occupational Therapists Specialist Section in Mental Health.

The study was a comparison study and used vignette (case summary) representations of clinical scenarios. Vignettes are well-recognised tools used in the determination of how clinical judgements in client care situations are made (Hughes & Huby, 2002; Ludwick & Zeller, 2001). They have previously been used in occupational therapy and mental health research (Harries & Gilhooly 2003b). From a research perspective they can be viewed as 'simulated clients' and bring the advantages of being able to manipulate their presentation and present the same 'client' to a number of different participants. For the purposes of this study, the vignettes were developed by a panel of 15 occupational therapists working in adult community mental health teams and were based on realistic clinical scenarios. A specific internet study site was created by a software consultant to conduct the study. Participants logged on to the site and were randomly assigned to one of two groups: case vignette alone or case vignette with a scored OCAIRS. They then completed 40 randomly presented vignettes (30 originals + 10 repeats). At the end of each vignette, participants were asked to prioritise the client's top three issues that, in their clinical judgement, were the most pressing. At the time of writing this chapter, data collection for this study is coming to an end and the final analysis has yet to be conducted. However, I hope that this study will be the first in a range of comparative studies that I will conduct to examine the different decision-making styles and strategies that therapists use in order to clarify, which are more effective in clinical practice.

Another important factor that was highlighted was the interdependence of clinicians and academics in conducting clinically relevant rigorous research. Conducting large-scale research projects is simply beyond the reach of an individual clinician. Equally, without clinical collaborators, the staff of research units cannot conduct meaningful research. Neither can fulfil a significant research function without the other. In this respect, clinical and academic partnerships that have been presented specifically within occupational therapy (Kielhofner, 2005; Crist *et al.*, 2005) and more generally at a policy level within nursing, midwifery and allied health professions in general (Scottish Executive, 2006) are clearly models of how the profession should build its research capacity and provide structures that can support clinicians, academics and the public to conduct rigorous research to improve the care and rehabilitation of clients.

My postdoctoral fellowship flew by, and I capitalised on this experience and funding to develop my skills in quantitative research methods and statistics to gain a greater knowledge of decision-making theories, to develop and submit grant applications and to submit peer-reviewed journal papers (Duncan & Nicol, 2004; Duncan *et al.*, 2006) and a research methods chapter (Duncan, 2006b) from my PhD thesis.

Towards the end of my fellowship, a permanent position arose within the unit for a clinical research fellow. This was another opportunity not to be missed. I applied for and was successful in gaining the post. As a clinical research fellow I am now leading a strand of work on judgement and decision making in mental health. It is an ideal position as it focuses on developing and leading on clinically relevant research projects in mental health, but such a position I could never have foreseen holding when I entered occupational therapy, or even when I commenced my doctoral studies.

Clarifying my research vision

Having taken my first faltering steps on a developing clinical–academic career pathway, I have now developed some clarity in vision about the shape and defining principles the of my future work and have developed some views about the shape of research that I believe occupational therapy in mental health, and in general, should follow if it is to achieve its goal of becoming an evidence-based profession.

First, I plan to focus on clinically relevant research that answers questions of direct patient relevance. This may seem an unnecessary statement, but a great deal of research has been carried out on issues of tangential relevance, and this not only fails to help the clients we work with but also impacts on the credibility of the profession. My second point relates to the epistemological position of my research. The nature of knowledge and what best constitutes evidence has generated a considerable amount of literature itself in healthcare and occupational therapy is no exception (Bannigan, 2002; Copley, 2002; Hyde, 2002, 2004; Legg & Walker, 2002;

Maclean & Jones, 2002; Bryant, 2004; Eva & Paley, 2004; Duncan & Nicol, 2004). Broadly speaking, all research falls within two scientific paradigms: scientific realism, which is the belief that the world has an existence that is separate to our perception of it (Williams & May, 1996), and scientific idealism, which believes the world is constructed and understood in the mind (Williams & Mays, 1996; Pope & Mays, 2000). The way researchers view these paradigms will strongly influence the direction of their research. I have argued (Duncan & Nicol, 2004) that neither of these positions is useful in occupational therapy research. Instead I have adopted a further perspective entitled subtle realism (Kirk Millar, 1986; Hammersley, 1992). Subtle realism suggests that most research involves subjective perceptions and observations and concedes that different methods will produce different pictures of the participants being studied. However, it also states that such perceptions and observations do not preclude the existence of independent phenomena and that objects, relationships and interventions can be studied and understood; the objective is the search for knowledge of which we can be reasonably confident (Murphy *et al.*, 1998). Whilst to some this position may appear to be epistemological fence sitting, to others (e.g. Hammersley, 1992; Murphy *et al.*, 1998) it seems the most valuable and pragmatic approach to health care research. Epistemological clarity is important, as a researcher's understanding of knowledge guides his or her selection of research methods.

Consequently, I view both qualitative and quantitative research methods as useful in the pursuit of knowledge. But, I firmly believe that the questions that require answering in mental health occupational therapy today are more suited to quantitative rather than qualitative methods. Qualitative methods undoubtedly have a place in the earlier stages of a study to define the problem, or in the later stages to clarify findings. However, without quantitative research of the effectiveness of occupational therapy interventions, they will continue to be missed from national clinical guidelines for best practice and therapists will continue to be pressured to work more generically in evidence-based interventions. As quantitative research is empirically based, it is inevitable that not all the findings that emerge will support our professional hypotheses. I believe that we have to become comfortable in recognising that not all occupational therapy interventions will be found to be effective. High-quality research will mean abandoning some of our practices, perhaps even those we closely cherish, as well as promoting those that are found to be more effective. But only in this way will clients benefit and it is for them, not the profession that we exist.

My final point is that there is a pressing need for comparative research within the profession. Many different theoretical models and frames of reference have been presented, developed and debated within occupational therapy, but rarely have these approaches been compared to determine which has the greatest clinical benefit. Now more than ever, there is a need to conduct research in this field. Without it, occupational therapy's days as a credible profession in mental health will be numbered. Conducting such research will, of course, not be simple. It will require complex research designs, for example, a cluster randomised control trial where departments instead of individuals are the unit of randomisation, and sophisti-cated statistical analyses, such as multi-level modelling that takes into account the various factors that can impact of care; from the therapist to the organisation. With the correct clinical–academic partnerships such studies are feasible and should be conducted.

An emerging pathway

When I first decided to pursue a clinical–academic/research career, I had little idea of the journey that lay ahead of me. Options at that time were limited and I simply imagined I would become an occupational therapy lecturer, which is a challenging enough post in itself. Recent years have witnessed the emergence of several clinical–academic routes and options are now increasing for therapists to undertake taught or research master's, PhDs or professional/clinical doctorates. A variety of post-doctoral opportunities are now developing. Professionally therapists can choose to remain based in clinical practice to develop their research expertise and collabo-rations or move to academia and take up a post in an increasing variety of lectur-ing and research positions. A variety of shared clinical–academic positions also exist. Clinical–academic careers are now being promoted at a policy level, bring-ing a new credibility to this career choice. There is, however, no single pathway. My ongoing clinical–academic career has taken many twists and turns, and I could never have foreseen how it would have unfolded to date at the beginning of my career. With the past being the best predictor of the future, it would be foolish indeed to predict what my future steps could be!

Summary

Reflecting on this, some key lessons that I have learn in the development of a clinical–academic career to date emerge:

■ Be proactive.
■ Build clinical and academic partnerships with a wide range of personnel and expertise.
■ Be open to all new opportunities as they arise.
■ Develop a thick skin in the face of rejection.
■ Be dogged in your determination to succeed.

New pathways are emerging for occupational therapists interested in pursuing a clinical–academic career. That this has occurred at all is due to the giants on whose shoulders we now stand – those leading therapists who have gone before us and made the way for occupational therapy a credible academic profession in mental health. It is up to us and those that follow us to ensure that the next steps are taken and their work was not in vain.

Questioning your Practice

1. What role do you want research to play in your professional career?
2. Who are the important people in your setting whom you could collaborate with so as to develop your research skills and expertise?
3. What research opportunities exist today that you could grasp?

References

Bannigan K (2002) EBP, RCTs and a climate of mutual respect. *British Journal of Occupational Therapy*, *65(8)*, (Letter), 391–392.

Bannigan K, Duncan EAS (2001) A Survey of post-registration research students in occupational therapy. *British Journal of Occupational Therapy*, *64(6)*, 278–284.

Blair SEE, Daniel MA (2006) An introduction to the psychodynamic frame of reference. In: EAS Duncan, ed. *Foundations for Practice in Occupational Therapy* (4th edn). Edinburgh: Elsevier/Churchill Livingstone, 233–254.

Bryant W (2004) Numbers in evidence.. *British Journal of Occupational Therapy*, *67(2)*, (Letter), 99–100.

Copley J (2002) RCTs: continuing the debate. *British Journal of Occupational Therapy*, *65(7)*, (letter) 346–347.

Crist P, Munoz JP, Hansen AW, *et al.* (2005) The Practice Scholar Program: an academic-practice partnership to promote the scholarship of 'best practices'. *Occupational Therapy in Health Care*, *19(1/2)*, 71–94.

Delamont S, Atkinson P, Parry O (1997) *Supervising the PhD: A Guide to Success.* Buckingham: Open University Press.

Donnelly JP, Guy S (1998) Evaluation of a first stage pilot project to address offending behaviour in a mentally disordered offender population in Scotland. *Psychiatric Care, 5(3)*, 106–108.

Donnelly JP, Scott MF (1999) Evaluation of an offending behaviour programme with a mentally disordered offender population. *British Journal of Forensic Practice, 1(4)*, 25–32.

Donnelly J, Williamson L, Duncan EAS (2001) Moral reasoning and empathy. *Forensic Update*, 6–7 October 2001, 5–11.

Duncan EAS (1999) Occupational therapy in mental health: it is time to recognise that it has come of age. *British Journal of Occupational Therapy, 62(11)*, 521–522.

Duncan EAS (2003a) Cognitive-behavioural therapy in Physiotherapy and Occupational Therapy. In: T Everett, M Donaghy, S Feaver (eds) *Interventions for Mental Health: An Evidence Based Approach.* Edinburgh: Butterworth Heinemann.

Duncan EAS (2003b) Sex offender Rehabilitation and the Role of the Occupational Therapist. In: L Couldrick, D Alred (eds) *Forensic Occupational Therapy.* London: London: Whurr Publications, 195–206.

Duncan EAS (2006a) The cognitive-behavioural frame of reference. In: EAS Duncan (ed.) (2005) *Foundations for Practice in Occupational Therapy* (4th edn). Edinburgh: Elsevier/Churchill Livingstone, 217–232.

Duncan EAS (2006b) The nature and use of consensus methodology in practice. In: G Kielhofner (ed.) *Scholarship in Occupational Therapy: Methods of Inquiry for Enhancing Practice.* Philadelphia, PA: F.A Davis, pp. 401–410.

Duncan EAS, ed. (2006c) *Foundations for Practice in Occupational Therapy* (4th edn). Edinburgh: Elsevier/ Churchill Livingstone.

Duncan EAS, Forsyth K, Ashby M, Summerfield-Mann L (2004) *Occupational Therapy Service Strategy 2003/2004: Promoting health, reducing risk and offending behaviour though everyday activity.* Carstairs: The State Hospitals Board for Scotland, Available at http://www.tsh.scot.nhs.uk/FreedomOfInformation/docs/Public%20Health/OT%20Strategy.pdf (last accessed 12 July 2007).

Duncan EAS, Moody K (2003) Integrated care pathways in mental health settings: An occupational therapy perspective. *British Journal of Occupational Therapy, 66(10)*, 473–478.

Duncan EAS, Munro K, Nicol M (2003) Research priorities in forensic occupational therapy. *British Journal of Occupational Therapy, 66(2)*, 55–64.

Duncan EAS, Nicol M (2004) Subtle reasoning and occupational therapy: an alternative approach to knowledge generation and evaluation. *British Journal of Occupational Therapy, 67(10)*, 453–456.

Duncan EAS, Nicol M, Ager A (2004) Factors that constitute a good cognitive behavioural treatment manual: A Delphi study. *Behavioural and Cognitive Psychotherapy, 32(2)*, 199–213.

Duncan EAS, Nicol M, Ager A, Dalgleish L (2006) A Systematic Review of Structured Group Interventions with Mentally Disordered Offenders. *Criminal Behaviour and Mental Health, 16(4)*, 217–241.

Duncan EAS, Thomson LDG, Short A (2000) Clinical guidelines within mental health services: an overview of the appraisal and implementation process. *British Journal of Occupational Therapy, 63(11)*, 557–560.

Eva G, Paley J (2004) Numbers in evidence. *British Journal of Occupational Therapy, 67(1)*, 47–50.

Forsyth K, Duncan EAS, Summerfield Mann L (2005a) Scholarship of practice in the United Kingdom: an occupational therapy service case study. *Occupational Therapy in Health Care, 19(1/2)*, 17–29.

Forsyth K, Walker K, Duncan EAS (2005b) Forensic occupational circumstances assessment interview and rating scale. In: K Forsyth, S Deshpande, G Kielhofner *et al. The Occupational Circumstances Assessment Interview and Rating Scale,* (OCAIRS) © Chicago, IL: University of Illinois, Model of Human Occupation Clearing House, 115–123.

Forsyth K, Parkinson S, Kielhofner G, Keller J, Summerfield Mann L, Duncan EAS *(Submitted)* The measurement properties of the Model of Human Occupation Screening Tool (MOHOST). *British Journal of Occupational Therapy.*

Fowler Davis S, Bannigan K (2000) Priorities in mental health research: the results of a live research project. *British Journal of Occupational Therapy, 63(3)*, 98–104.

Fowler Davis S, Hyde P (2002) Priorities in mental health research: an update. *British Journal of Occupational Therapy, 65(8)*, 387–389.

Freemantle N (1996) Are decisions taken by health care professionals rational? A non systematic review of experimental and quasi-experimental literature. *Health Policy, 38(2)*, 71–81.

Grove WM, Meehl PE (1996) Comparative efficiency of informal (subjective, impressionistic) and formal (mechanical, algorithmic) prediction procedures: The clinical/statistical controversy. *Psychology, Public Policy, and Law, 2(2)*, 1–31.

Hammersley M (1992) *What's Wrong with Ethnography?* London: Routledge.

Harries PA, Gilhooly K (2003a) Generic and specialist occupational therapy casework in community mental health teams. *British Journal of Occupational Therapy, 66(3)*, 101–109.

Harries PA, Gilhooly K (2003b) Identifying occupational therapists' referral priorities in community health. *Occupational Therapy International, 10(2)*, 150–164.

Holloway I, Walker J (2000) *Getting a PhD in Health and Social Care.* Oxford: Blackwell Publishing.

Hughes R, Huby M (2002) The application of vignettes in social and nursing research. *Journal of Advanced Nursing, 37(4)*, 382.

Hyde P (2002) RCTs: legitimate research tool or fancy mathematics? *British Journal of Occupational Therapy, 65(9),* (Letter), 435–36.

Hyde P (2004) Fool's gold: examining the use of gold standards in the production of research evidence. *British Journal of Occupational Therapy, 67(2),* 89–93.

Ingram G (2003) Play and occupational therapy, In: T Everett, M Donaghy, S Feaver (eds) *Interventions for Mental Health: An Evidence Based Approach.* Edinburgh: Butterworth Heinemann, pp.185–195.

Kielhofner G (2005) A scholarship of practice: creating discourse between theory, research and practice. *Occupational Therapy in Health Care, 19(1/2),* 7–16.

Kirk J, Miller M (1986) *Reliability and Validity in Qualitative Research.* Newbury Park: Sage.

Legg L, Walker M (2002) Let us use randomised controlled trials. *British Journal of Occupational Therapy, 65(3)* (Letter), 149.

Ludwick R, Zeller RA (2001) The Factorial Survey: An experimental Method to replicate Real World Problems. *Nursing Research, 50(2),* 129.

MacLean F, Jones D (2002) RCTs: need for wider debate. *British Journal of Occupational Therapy, 65(6),* (letter), 294–295.

Mental Welfare Commission (2000) *Mental Welfare Commission for Scotland: Annual Report 1999–2000.* Edinburgh: Mental Welfare Commission.

Murphy E, Dingwall R, Greatbatch D, Parker S, Watson P (1998) Qualitative research methods in health technology assessment: a review of the literature. *Health Technology Assessment, 2 (16),* 2.

Pope C, Mays N (2000) Qualitative Methods in Health Research. In: C Pope, N Mays (eds) *Qualitative Research in Health Care* (2nd edn). London: British Medical Journal Publishing Group, 1–10.

Scottish Executive (2004) *Allied Health Professions Research and Development Action Plan.* Edinburgh: The Scottish Executive.

Scottish Executive (2006) *Delivering Care, Enabling health.* Edinburgh: The Scottish Executive. The State Hospitals Board for Scotland (2002) *Annual Report 2001-2002.* Carstairs: The State Hospital.

Urquhart G (2002) Setting up a forensic occupational therapy service. In: L Couldrick, D Alred (eds) *Forensic Occupational Therapy.* London: Whurr, pp. 117–125.

Williams M, May T (1996) *Introduction to the Philosophy of Social Research.* London: UCL Press.

14 Researching within mental health
Slow and steady – a Canadian tour

Thelma Sumsion

Personal narrative

The journey to my current position has been rather tortoise like, just slow and steady. It began in the summer before my last year in high school with a job in a large mental health facility. This was my introduction to occupational therapy and I learned that it really suited me. I grew up on in a farming community where people mattered, and here was a profession where I could work with people by engaging them in tasks that kept them happy and occupied. This is not the major focus of the profession we know today, but it was so in the late 1960s. The first step of my education began with a move to the big city (there is another story in that adventure) and the completion of a diploma in physical and occupational therapy. The tortoise-like progress to my present position was underway and I moved slowly forward to a BSc (Occupational Therapy) 10 years later, and a master's degree in education 4 years after that. The education piece of my story finally concluded with the completion of my PhD in 2003. Along the way I worked in a variety of mental health programmes with many client groups and in a number of different positions including therapist, manager, consultant and educator, both in Canada and England, and now as the director of a school of occupational therapy in a research-intensive university in Canada. My current research focuses on client-centred practice with people with severe and persistent mental illness, as I am convinced that this approach really does matter to this population and makes a significant impact on the quality of the interventions in which they engage. I have learned many valuable lessons during this journey that has spanned close to 40 years. Most of those lessons have come from the clients, and it is for them that I write this chapter.

Introduction

Throughout my career I have tried to follow the advice of Paulo Coelho (1988). He writes about dreams and that the only thing that makes them impossible to achieve is the fear of failure and the only way to learn is through action. However, it took me a while to incorporate these wise words into my professional life. Initially, I was a research phobic who was afraid of failure and would rather teach, work with clients and do administrative tasks than engage in research. However, I gradually came to understand that, like it or not, I was engaging in research on a daily basis. I did not have big research grants, and at this initial stage, I was not publishing but I was asking questions, the point where any research project begins. Some examples of these questions include the following: What was important to the clients with whom I worked? What were the approaches I used that elicited the best responses? What led up to the breakthroughs that made such a difference to the clients? At this stage in the journey I noticed that often the therapeutic outcomes were not directly attributable to what I did but more to how I did it. I was being a client-centred therapist and I realised it was time to take action. I wanted to know a lot more about this approach and why it seemed to make a difference.

The Canadian tour – the early days

Client-centred practice did not originate in occupational therapy, nor is it unique to our profession. However, we are leaders in this approach with particular emphasis in the area of mental health. The concept first appeared through the work of Carl Rogers (1939) when he outlined an approach that was non-directive and focused on concerns expressed by the individual client (Law, 1998). Canadian therapists were fortunate to have an opportunity to build on this work and that of Reed and Sanderson (1980) through a national taskforce jointly funded by the Canadian Association of Occupational Therapists (CAOT) and the Department of National Health and Welfare (DNHW). I had the privilege of chairing this group that consisted of occupational therapists from across Canada who worked in a range of areas of practice, as well as medical representatives. We worked together to produce several documents including *Guidelines for the Client-Centred Practice of Occupational Therapy* (DNHW & CAOT, 1983), *Intervention Guidelines for the Client-Centred Practice of Occupational Therapy* (DNHW & CAOT, 1986) and *Toward Outcome Measures in Occupational Therapy* (DNHW & CAOT, 1987).These documents introduced therapists to the concept of client-centred practice and the processes and procedures necessary for its implementation. The funding organisations asked the taskforce in which area of practice it would be most difficult to apply these concepts, and the overwhelming response was mental health. I am not convinced the answer to that question would be the same today, but that was the view in the early 1990s. As a result a subgroup of the main taskforce, along with some additional therapists, worked on the production of the publication titled *Occupational Therapy Guidelines for Client-Centred Mental Health Practice* (DNHW & CAOT, 1993). This document interpreted and applied the generic guidelines, from the original documents, to practice in mental health. Client-centred practice is not clearly defined as a distinct entity but there is a considerable amount of direction to therapists regarding how the approach should be applied, including the following:

■ this approach refers to practice in which client's experiences and knowledge are central and carry authority within the client–professional partnership (p. 5);

■ occupational therapists have an ethical and moral responsibility to ensure that clients are as informed as possible of the options and risks associated with possible courses of action (p. 5); and

■ a client-centred approach requires occupational therapists to actively seek and structure opportunities for clients to have real choices and authority commensurate with their skills and experience (p. 5).

However, concerns have been raised that having all of these nationally created and approved guidelines has not necessarily made us consistent and effective client-centred therapists. Ten years after the launch of the first national document, I was concerned that therapists did not clearly understand the implications of the proposed model on their practice. Were we truly involving the client as the decision maker in all stages of the therapeutic process? Were we ready to relinquish some of the power that this involvement might require? Were we clearly defining who the client was before we engaged in the process (Sumsion, 1993)? Unfortunately, the honest answer to these questions was 'no' at that time and in some ways is still 'no' today. Rebeiro (2001a) subsequently reiterated some of these same concerns and added an enlightened view by stating that ' by remembering the person, all that they were, are and can be, client-centred practice can help to bridge disability and illness with hope, instead of despair' (p. 66).

Moving forward

Many committed therapists/researchers have taken the initial work and concerns forward to enable a deeper understanding of the importance of applying a client-centred approach in mental health. Townsend (1998), a member of the original taskforce, continued to lead the way through publishing her critique on empowerment in the organisation of mental health services. Her work clearly showed that many aspects of a client-centred approach were not being applied. Instead, organisations were controlling decisions hierarchically, preserving exclusion and managing cases rather than working with the individual to design unique solutions. All of these issues conflict with a client-centred focus that supports consumer involvement in decisions, inclusion and an individual approach. Next, Corring and Cook (1999) examined the client's perspective and found, in support of Roger's original premise, that it is important for clients to be viewed as valuable human beings. In their study, clients spoke openly about the negative attitudes of the service providers, their superficial knowledge of clients, their use of techniques that did not meet the client's needs and the importance of valuing the clients' experiences and taking time to talk. Rebeiro is also an important contributor to this discussion (see more of her work in Chapter 8). The clients that she interviewed stressed the importance of choice, a focus on them as individuals rather than on the illness and inclusion in the decision-making process (Rebeiro, 2000). Her subsequent work reinforced the findings of Corring and Cook (1999) as the clients in her study wanted to be involved in environments that affirmed they were people of worth (Rebeiro, 2001b).

These researchers have raised consistent, important issues that are fundamental to client-centred practice, including engaging with clients as individuals, taking time to get to know these individuals and enabling their choice of intervention.

My contributions to the journey

My involvement in the guidelines project spanned more than 15 years. Throughout that time I continued to work in a variety of roles in the mental health system and endeavoured to apply the concepts we were discussing, writing and explaining to other therapists. I certainly experienced the challenges firsthand but wanted to know more about these issues. It was time to become a serious researcher. My opportunity to do so came in 1996, when I moved to London. I was teaching at Brunel University and I was offered the opportunity to engage in PhD studies. Here was the chance to build on my Canadian experiences, really delve into client-centred practice and come to grips with its many challenging components. This phase of the journey covered 5 years and allowed me to engage therapists throughout the UK in many phases of a process to clearly define client-centred practice. There were Canadian definitions (Law *et al.*, 1995; CAOT, 2002), but I wanted to contribute a consensus definition that truly incorporated the views of therapists working in differing geographical areas as well as a wide range of areas of practice. The research process incorporated a range of methods including the Delphi Technique, the Nominal Group Technique within a focus-group format, consensus meetings and interviews. This was an exciting journey in itself and the destination was reached through the creation of the following preamble to and definition of client-centred practice:

Preamble

There are many factors that influence the successful implementation of client-centred practice including a clear determination of who the client is and the recognition of the impact of resources.

Definition

Client-centred occupational therapy is a partnership between the client and the therapist that empowers the client to engage in functional performance and fulfil his or her occupational roles in a variety of environments. The client participates actively in negotiating goals that are given priority and are at the centre of assessment, intervention and evaluation. Throughout the process the therapist listens to and respects the client's values, adapts the interventions to meet the client's needs and enables the client to make informed decisions (Sumsion, 2000).

This definition echoes many of the important issues identified by the previous researchers referred to in this chapter, including forming partnerships with clients, engaging them throughout the therapeutic process and enabling informed decisions.

At this point in my research journey I had a more in-depth understanding of the components of client-centred practice and therapists' views of these. However, I had no idea if this definition had any clinical applicability. The final phase of the study enabled me to take this definition into an out-patient mental health setting and conduct in-depth interviews with therapists about the barriers to and opportunities for its application. This was a positive experience, and I wanted to clone this group of therapists as they were truly client-centred and readily demonstrated the components of the definition. They challenged the system to enable clients to reach their goals by responding to the clients' issues, juggling the reason for the referral, adapting interventions and providing relevant information. They did encounter barriers such as time, power struggles and cultural road blocks, but they worked with the client to overcome all of these (Sumsion, 2004).

However, I was aware that in many ways I was being a hypocrite as I was studying client-centred practice but had not yet involved the clients. Therefore, some initial interviews were undertaken to determine their views of the definition in relation to barriers to and opportunities for its implementation. It was clear that client-centred practice was important to this group and that they valued the information they were given to enable choices. They wanted to participate in determining goals, but to do so they had to overcome fear and issues presented by the severity of their illness (Sumsion, 2005). Overall, it appeared that the concepts presented in the definition including partnership, empowerment, active engagement, listening, adapting and enabling were important to both therapists and clients, but there was still more work to be done. During this time I also edited an initial book that was revised in 2006, to help therapists more clearly understand issues related to implementation with various client groups (Sumsion, 2006).

At this point the journey takes a slight pause as I decided to return to Canada. Once I was settled and had the challenges of my new position in some perspective, I undertook a project to replicate the final phases of the work completed in England to see if there were any similarities in the two countries in relation to the opportunities for and barriers to the application of this approach from the perspective of both therapists and clients. This work has been completed but not yet published. However, initial findings certainly do indicate many similarities. Canadian therapists also stressed the importance of enabling choice by not making decisions for the clients, explaining the likely outcome of various choices and enabling clients to have a say or at least some input into the decisions that affect them. It was felt to be impossible to work with the clients without effective rapport. These therapists also stated that it was wonderful to get to know the clients in a way that enabled them to become truly comfortable with the therapist. They recognised the importance of working in a partnership with the client with the therapists telling them what they could offer and listening to the clients' needs and wants. They described this true partnership as one that meant equal kinds of responsibility and commitment. These therapists also accepted that they had to broaden their horizons to encompass the clients' interests, look at the big picture and enable them to set and achieve their goals. The clients in this study expressed that the programme in which they were engaged fostered a culture of respect, empowered them, was flexible enough to ensure their needs were met and created an atmosphere of care and partnership.

Barriers

I am confident that any therapist who has attempted to implement a client-centred approach in a mental health setting could list the barriers that were encountered. However, there is some literature to which we can refer for clarification, or perhaps affirmation, of these challenges. Sumsion and Smyth (2000) found that the therapist and client having differing goals was the barrier that most prevented the implementation of a client-centred approach. The therapist's attitudes, beliefs and values and the culture in the employment environment also posed formidable challenges. Wilkins *et al.* (2001) concluded, from the amalgamation of data from three different studies, that there were challenges presented by the system, such as support for the implementation of a client-centred approach, by the therapist, including the required transition from paternalism to sharing and partnership, and by the client, through the recognition that some client groups will be more receptive to this approach than others.

Throughout my professional career I have certainly encountered many of these barriers, but I confess to being one who frequently ignored them or tried my best to work around them. But, this is not always a successful strategy. In the early days of my career I worked on an adolescent in-patient unit. I tried valiantly to apply a client-centred approach but struggled to find a meaningful activity in which the clients would willingly engage. Finally, we settled on a car wash, which seemed to me to be a reasonably safe and productive activity. We agreed on the responsibility of the members of this partnership. The adolescents would decide on a date, make the advertising posters and, as only adolescents can, harass the staff to ensure their cars were all lined up. I was to secure the necessary equipment and obtain permission from the administration of the hospital. The sad outcome was that, no matter what I tried, including official memos, begging and pleading, I could not get the administration to approve this activity. They were very concerned about safety, including falls, and potential damage to vehicles. I tried for weeks, but in the end the activity did not occur as the environment had presented a barrier I could not overcome. I was left to deal with a renewed ambivalence among the client group and my own frustration at not meeting my obligations as a member of the partnership. We did work it through and were able to philosophically examine the lessons that were learned, but there is no doubt that the partnership experienced a significant setback. Some years later, a psychiatrist, who always seemed to get approval for every programme, taught me that it was easier to ask for forgiveness than permission, and perhaps that is a strategy I should have applied.

I learned other valuable lessons in this position. Almost 40 years later I still remember a young man with whom I worked very closely and with whom a client-centred approach was working very well. He came from a disadvantaged background and his goal was to complete his high school education. He worked very hard, and as his discharge date approached, we worked on strategies to help him face the obvious environmental challenges he would encounter in the community, such as not having a quiet place to study and friends who would try to entice him to engage in illegal activities rather than completing his school work. This latter situation should have triggered the realisation that he was returning to a large environment that did not support educational pursuits. Had the Canadian Model of Occupational Performance (CAOT, 2002) been integrated into my practice at this time, I would have clearly understood the importance of environmental issues. Then, I focused on the smaller issues and failed to see the big picture. Ultimately, he was not successful in reaching his goals in the community, which was, in part, attributable to my narrow focus. The lesson learned here was that a client-centred approach has to take place within the realities of the physical, social and cultural environments. The positive aspect of this phase of my experience was that I worked with a terrific team on this unit who were primarily client-centred. They went the extra mile to ensure client needs were understood and addressed and programmes were designed to allow the clients to achieve their goals, including education.

I also tried to implement the principles of client-centred practice in my work as a consultant. This role took me into the remote parts of northern Ontario where therapists worked with a range of client groups including those experiencing severe and persistent mental disorders. There was considerable variation in the number of accessible community resources, including those locations that were well served and those who were left to fend for themselves. I worked with these therapists to help them determine the priority issues, outline the available resources and, in some cases, determine a lobbying strategy. Here was a strong example of providing relevant information, within a different type of partnership, to enable choices that were frequently rather limited. There was also a clear requirement for the use of creativity, which, although not a documented element, is a strong component of client-centred practice if desired goals are to be achieved.

In my role as a manager in a large mental health facility and, today, in an academic department, I have also tried to practise what I was preaching. One of my main roles in these positions was to remove barriers so goals could be reached. Examples include starting new programmes that met an identified client need in times when programmes were being cut due to financial restraints; seizing opportunities to launch new graduate programmes to enable academic staff to have student supervisory experience; and helping academic staff to set priorities and give up historical practices so the age-old issue of not enough time could be addressed.

Time is definitely a major barrier to client-centred practice. However, my plea is that we just accept the fact that there is never enough time to do everything we either need or want to do in both our personal and professional lives. I think society would be much happier if we stopped beating ourselves up about this fact and just got on with it. Yes, it does take more time initially to engage in a client-centred process as we need to really understand the clients' stories to enable us to help them set goals within a context that is meaningful to them. Once this engagement has occurred and they are working toward these meaningful goals, they will require less input from us. So, in the long run, this approach does not take more time (Sumsion, 2006). In support of this, Stewart (2003) found 19 articles that addressed the question of time and reported that the conclusions were inconsistent. These varied from no difference in the amount of time required to those that did take longer as this approach resulted in the discussion of a larger number of issues.

I have learned many lessons from all of the people I have worked with, but it is the clients who have taught me the most valuable ones. Through my research I continue to be involved with a community programme for people with severe and persistent mental illness. This is definitely client-centred as all of the groups and activities are based around issues that the clients have raised. A client council oversees the programme that is run primarily by occupational therapists, and there is great diversity in what is offered, from music groups to a café and catering business, to discussion groups where problems are addressed. The clients choose the programmes in which they want to be involved. I recently attended a talent show that was organised by the clients and staff at this programme. People exhibited a wide range of talents from singing, playing musical instruments, reading poetry and displaying art and crafts. The room was full of people, and these clients, who were coping with a range of symptoms, stood up and shared their talents to thunderous applause. I do not know how you get much more client-centred than that as they were the focus of this programme and were being supported to meet this particular goal. The talent was quite varied, but the enthusiasm and courage was unanimous. These clients have taught me that adversity can be overcome and that, with the right encouragement and support, they can achieve their goals. Some of these clients have also willingly come into university and freely told their stories so that occupational therapy students can understand the many personal and environmental challenges they have overcome. Again, what courage! I often wonder if I would have the courage to face the adversities they have tackled. Would I be able to deal with the symptoms of an illness that I know will never go away? Would I be able to handle the loss of family and friends who cannot understand what I am experiencing? How would I deal with stigma expressed by a community that chooses not to incorporate me into their activities? So, for me the bottom line is that these people are to be admired and welcomed as teachers and colleagues. A client-centred approach enables all of us to include them in the programmes we are there to offer and to ensure that those they are clearly meeting identified needs. They face more daily barriers than I will ever face; so it is my responsibility to work in partnership with them to remove their barriers and advocate for the inclusion and achievement of their goals.

Still work to do

Recently, I attended a multi-disciplinary conference that was focused on client-centred practice and on ethical issues related to client-centred practice. Both included issues related to mental health, although that was not their primary focus. I also attend numerous sessions at local and national occupational therapy conferences with client-centred practice in the session title. I usually come away from these experiences asking myself if the presenters really understood what being client-centred meant – they simply failed to convey that understanding clearly as the right words were there but the actions taken were not truly client-centred. It is very difficult to be a client-centred therapist. It is hard to take the time to really understand the person's story, to discuss realities related to goals, to advocate and/or remove barriers so those goals can be achieved, and to address safety, and not to let risks and fear of failure prevent your support of the chosen goals. Much more work needs to be done on all levels to really understand and activate issues related to power sharing, listening and communicating, making true partnerships work and enabling choice (Sumsion & Law, 2006). Overall, the clients I have spoken to tell me that we need to work on not taking away their hope, not being afraid to let them fail and enabling them to at least work toward their goals.

Final thoughts

The invitation to write this chapter has provided me with an exciting opportunity to reflect on the connection between client-centred practice and my career. The conclusion I have reached is that it is very difficult to be a client-centred therapist. It means giving and asking a lot of yourself and being strong enough to carry on when the challenges for implementing this way of working seem simply insurmountable. If you are not truly interested in people, then you cannot be a client-centred therapist. You have to really want to know their stories as it is not good enough to know that you should do that from an academic perspective. You have to be willing to understand and appreciate the complexities of living with a mental illness. Rejection, avoidance, pain and suffering are all very real for this client group. You need to really care about them as people, learn what makes them tick and what is important to them.

Another word of caution regarding taking a client-centred approach relates to what I call the 'opening-the-door factor'. You will not find any literature about this, but I have certainly learned that if I open the client-centred door with my clients, I have to be prepared to engage with whatever walks through. I cannot build rapport, engage in a partnership with them, and then be frightened off by an issue they raise that is important to them. Therefore, I really need to know myself and my comfort and confidence levels so I can engage, and perhaps redirect, but not be shocked and walk away. What am I prepared to engage in and what is outside of my comfort level? Personally, I know that I cannot work with people who have consciously physically abused others. I know I do not handle interactions with this client group well. I have tried to be open with my team about this and will redirect clients, who certainly deserve a meaningful interaction with a caring team member, to the person who can work comfortably with them.

I have worked with client-centred practice for a great many years and I am still learning about the complexities of this approach. Some of my failures still haunt me, but I have tried to learn from them to ensure I am offering my clients the best interaction possible. You can do the same.

Summary

My research journey built slowly to a climax, but my amazement at the courage of the clients with whom I work has only gained in strength. My final plea is that, as talented occupational therapists working in mental health settings, we accept the challenge of working in a client-centred way; that we commit ourselves to this approach and do whatever we can, no matter how small the effort may appear, to overcome the barriers that are presented by the system, ourselves and the clients. We can truly listen. We can ensure the clients' goals are incorporated into the plan that is hopefully being designed with them rather than for them. We can let them take risks, as that is how we all learn.

Questioning your Practice

1. How can I implement a more client-centred approach into my practice?
2. Do I create and/or support unnecessary barriers that prohibit the effective implementation of a client-centred approach?
3. Do I enable the clients to teach me valuable lessons as our partnership develops?

References

Canadian Association of Occupational Therapists (2002) *Enabling Occupation: An Occupational Therapy Perspective*. Ottawa: CAOT Publications ACE.

Coelho P (1988) *The Alchemist*. London: Thorsons.

Corring D, Cook J (1999) Client-centred care means that I am a valued human being. *Canadian Journal of Occupational Therapy, 66(2)*, 71–82.

Department of National Health and Welfare, Canadian Association of Occupational Therapists (1983) *Guidelines for the Client-Centred Practice of Occupational Therapy*. Ottawa: DNHW.

Department of National Health and Welfare, Canadian Association of Occupational Therapists (1986) *Intervention Guidelines for the Client-Centred Practice of Occupational Therapy*. Ottawa: DNHW.

Department of National Health and Welfare, Canadian Association of Occupational Therapists (1987) *Toward Outcome Measure in Occupational Therapy*. Ottawa: DNHW.

Department of National Health and Welfare, Canadian Association of Occupational Therapists (1993) *Occupational Therapy Guidelines for Client-Centred Mental Health Practice*. Ottawa: CAOT Publications ACE.

Law M (1998) *Client-Centered Occupational Therapy*. Thorofare, NJ: Slack.

Law M, Baptiste S, Mills J (1995) Client-centred practice: what does it mean and does it make a difference? *Canadian Journal of Occupational Therapy, 62(5)*, 250–257.

Rebeiro KL (2000) Client perspectives on occupational therapy practice: are we truly client-centred? *Canadian Journal of Occupational Therapy, 67(1)*, 7–14.

Rebeiro KL (2001a) Client-centred practice: body, mind and spirit resurrected. *Canadian Journal of Occupational Therapy, 68(2)*, 65–69.

Rebeiro, KL (2001b) Enabling occupation: the importance of an affirming environment. *Canadian Journal of Occupational Therapy, 68(2)*, 80–89.

Reed K, Sanderson SR (1980) *Concepts of Occupational Therapy*. Baltimore, MD: Williams & Wilkins.

Rogers CR (1939) *The Clinical Treatment of the Problem Child*. Boston, MA: Houghton-Mifflin.

Stewart M (2003) Questions about patient-centered care: answers from qualitative research. In: M Stewart, J Belle Brown, W Weston, IR McWhinney, CL McWIlliam, TR Freeman (eds) *Patient-Centered Medicine: Transforming the Clinical Method*. Abingdon: Radcliffe Medical Press Ltd.

Sumsion T (1993) Client-centred practice: the true impact. *Canadian Journal of Occupational Therapy, 60(1)*, 6–8.

Sumsion T (2000) A revised occupational therapy definition of client-centred practice. *British Journal of Occupational Therapy, 63(7)*, 304–309.

Sumsion T (2004) Pursuing the client's goals really paid off. *British Journal of Occupational Therapy, 67(1)*, 2–9.

Sumsion T (2005) Facilitating client-centred practice: insights from clients. *Canadian Journal of Occupational Therapy, 72(1)*, 13–20.

Sumsion T (2006) *Client-Centred Practice in Occupational Therapy: A Guide to Implementation*. (2nd edn). Edinburgh: Churchill Livingstone.

Sumsion T, Law M (2006) A review of evidence on the conceptual elements informing client-centred practice. *Canadian Journal of Occupational Therapy, 73(3)*, 153–162.

Sumsion T, Smyth G (2000) Barriers to client-centredness and their resolution. *Canadian Journal of Occupational Therapy, 67(1)*, 17–21.

Townsend E (1998) *Good Intentions Overruled: A Critique of Empowerment in the Routine Organization of Mental Health Services*. Toronto: University of Toronto Press.

Wilkins S, Pollock N, Rochon S, Law M (2001) Implementing client-centred practice: why is it so difficult to do? *Canadian Journal of Occupational Therapy, 68(2)*, 70–79.

15 Future prospects for occupational therapy in mental health

Christine Craik

Personal narrative

My career as an occupational therapist in mental health has several links with the earliest days of the profession in the UK. It has continued through my practising in mental health, developing and managing services, and then later teaching students about mental health, and now research (Craik & Pieris, 2006). I have also been involved in developing national policy in the UK and shaping the future of the profession in mental health (Craik *et al.*, 1998). From these experiences, I am in the fascinating position of being able to look back to the pioneers of the profession and see their influence on current practice and look forward to the challenges of the future in the knowledge that our heritage as a profession has a firm foundation and has survived and prospered through difficult times.

The influences on me have been my family and my Scottish heritage. Like many other people, I have become intrigued by my family history. I am fortunate that my parents, now both in their nineties, have clear memories of their childhood and of their family history and are happy to recount these.

My great-grandmother was left a widow with two young sons when her husband, a railway worker, was killed in an accident at work. As she lived in cottage owned by the railway company, she also lost her home. Well before the times of the welfare state, she had to support herself and her sons; so she moved to Glasgow and entered domestic service as a dairy maid. Her sons spent time in the stables, an interest that later developed into their future jobs as coachmen. However, in the early years of the twentieth century, my grandfather, realising that the days of horse-drawn transport were numbered and that the future was in motor cars, learned to drive and to work with cars. So he became the second chauffer in a grand Victorian house in Glasgow. It was here that my father, as a child of three in 1912, remembers being left in the care of his father to help in the garage, polishing the cars, when his mother took his younger sisters out. This interest in cars led to his apprenticeship and early career as a motor mechanic.

As was the custom in the 1920s and 1930s, my parents both left school and started work when they were 14 years old. But like most Scots, they valued education and were determined that their child would have the educational opportunities they were denied. Fortunately, I seem to have inherited their intelligence, and so I was able to benefit from these opportunities. I have also inherited their exemplification of the Scottish virtues of diligence, determination and making the most of what you have and not wasting time lamenting about what you do not have. These are the attributes that I have taken in to my professional life. I would also like to think that I have inherited my grandfather's instinct of knowing when something has had it day and it is time to move on. My parents have always been supportive of my career and have been interested in the writing of this chapter and on reading it in draft; my mother was able to suggest improvements to my grammar.

My first contact with occupational therapy in mental health was as a prospective student when I visited an occupational therapy department prior to attending a selection interview at the Glasgow School of Occupational Therapy. I went to a psychiatric unit within a general hospital, which had a large occupational therapy unit and associated day hospital. Farndale (1961), in his account of the day hospital movement, describes the building and its facilities, confirming my memory of it. I do not remember meeting patients on my visit, but I do recall the therapists' explanations not of what was being done but why. My account on returning home was that everything I had seen had a purpose beyond the obvious; I was entranced and I still am. I obtained a place at the Glasgow School of Occupational Therapy, where I was an average student – my main claim to fame was that I was the youngest in my year, starting the course when I was seventeen and a half and graduating and starting work as a therapist when I was just over 20 years of age.

My first post in mental health was at Gartnavel Royal Hospital in Glasgow. Here, in 1919, Dr David Henderson established occupational therapy in the UK and employed Dorothea Robertson as the first occupational instructor (Wilcock, 2002). With a distinguished beginning, the occupational therapy service was at an interesting stage in its development when I arrived, and I was able to contribute to it. Although the original building where the profession started was used as a ward, several years later the occupational therapy department relocated there. Thus, I worked for several years in the building where occupational therapy in the UK began.

But it is people more than places that make history; and I was fortunate to meet Margaret Barr Fulton, the first qualified occupational therapist to work in the UK. I first met Peg, as she was known, in 1982, when I sat next to her at a dinner to celebrate the Golden Jubilee of occupational therapy, when she recounted stories of Dr David Henderson and the early days of the profession. Later when I worked in Aberdeen, I met her again and I was conscious of her legacy of working for almost 40 years in mental health at the Royal Cornhill Hospital. With these connections with the beginning of the profession, I have been fortunate in the times in which I have worked as an occupational therapist. And if I have inherited my grandfather's ability to know when things have had their day, then occupational therapy has not.

Introduction

The purpose of this chapter is to predict the future of occupational therapy in mental health. But as with all attempts at prophesy, it is fraught with difficulties.

If an optimistic stance is taken and the events do not turn out as anticipated, then the opportunity for improvement has been lost. Equally, if a pessimistic view is taken, then the opportunity for additional growth may be lost. Striving to find a realistic position is the aim, but this chapter is structured to look at the optimistic and the pessimistic.

Best practice

Within the chapters of this book there have been examples of the very best occupational therapy in mental health. Evidence-based practice combined with imagination has moved the boundaries of the profession beyond its traditional precincts of institutions to enrich the lives of people with mental health problems living in the community. The scope of occupational therapy has been demonstrated from enabling people to engage in productive occupations that provide paid or voluntary employment to encouraging the development of artistic endeavours that promote self-esteem, from the application of narrative as a means of understanding people to the development of recovery as a vehicle to assist their rehabilitation and participation in their communities.

Research studies, relevant to occupational therapy and occupational science undertaken by occupational therapists and others, have been presented and the encouraging research careers of occupational therapists have been portrayed as examples for others. The research described has been relevant and practical, conducted with, and for, service users and providing the basis for further studies. There are indications, from the study of occupational science, that understanding the engagement of people in occupations that have meaning for them has implications for individuals and society in general.

All this is positive and bodes well for an optimistic and healthy future for occupational therapy. However, not everything is positive; contained within the chapters there are portents of unease. Although there are welcome developments in research in occupational therapy, there are indications that, until large-scale randomised controlled trials demonstrate the effectiveness of occupational therapy, the current small-scale, mainly qualitative studies, will not be accorded the same status. This is likely to have implications for the financing of services as evidence of the effectiveness of interventions will be required in the future. The move towards generic working is not universally welcomed. There are genuine concerns that the ethos of occupational therapy may be lost in the move to all mental health staff working in the same way and that the creativity and passion, that are the hallmark of occupational therapy, may be subsumed in a collective rush to the mediocre. There are signs, in several countries, that funding of occupational therapy may be restricted to focus exclusively on providing specific intervention and that this may curtail the ability of the profession to develop to its full potential though research and imaginative developments. There are obvious synergies between the drive to promote the social inclusion of people with mental health problems and the philosophy of occupational therapy. But if the profession does not rise to the current political imperative to address social inclusion, then others will do so. From one perspective this may not matter as the overriding obligation is that the needs of services users are addressed. However, there are indications that service users appreciate the approach of occupational therapy; so it would be negligent of the profession to overlook this important area.

Optimism or pessimism?

So, looking at these prospects for the profession in mental health, occupational therapists have, perhaps for a short period, an opportunity to influence its future. It must be acknowledged that the motivation for doing this is not professional self-promotion but a genuine and firmly held belief that occupational therapy has a major contribution to make to improve the lives of people with mental health problems. While the evidence base for this assertion would not meet the criteria for the highest levels of evidence, as expert opinion, it is, nevertheless, evidence.

International perspectives

The implications of the internationalisation of health care and of occupational therapy are having a profound impact on the profession. Throughout the world, there is an expansion in the movement of people from country to country, resulting in increased multi-cultural societies, and thus cultural awareness and sensitivity are essential to the delivery of contemporary occupational therapy. However, occupational therapy in mental health has developed at different rates in different countries as is demonstrated by the number of practitioners working in this area of practice throughout the world. If this is used as a crude measure of the influence of the profession, then the UK, with a high percentage of occupational therapists working in mental health, has the opportunity, and responsibility, to lead developments. That is not to devalue the contribution of others, quite the contrary; but the critical mass of occupational therapists working in mental health in the UK has the potential to make a significant impact. It will be important for the future to monitor the numbers of therapists in different countries, and national associations have a key function in doing this.

Individual and collective action to advance practice

This topic of this book is advanced practice and it contains many examples of the different ways in which this can be achieved. In recounting their narratives and describing their practice, the contributors have shared their professional identity and values, which, when taken together, provide a vivid picture of the best of current occupational therapy in mental health. In writing their chapters, the contributors have further advanced their own practice as the act of reflecting on their work, reading relevant literature, synthesising ideas and explaining them to others, which are conscious activities that reinforce good practice. The contributors have been prepared to expose their ideas, procedures and aspirations to scrutiny to advance the practice of others.

Reading literature is an essential part of this process, and therapists reading this book have engaged in a vital action in advancing their own practice, but more is required than reading. Identifying what occupational therapists can do both individually and, probably more importantly, through their collaboration with, and influence on, others will be an important step in advancing practice.

Continuing professional development

Advanced practice requires advanced thinking. While it is possible to achieve this in isolation, most people require stimulation, support and external motivation to do this. It is unlikely that individuals can become advanced practitioners without some further education or skills training. Perhaps in previous generations some occupational therapists could successfully undertake their pre-registration education and then rely on just doing the job to develop their skills sufficiently. But, even in the early days of practice, some therapists undertook further study. Wilcock (2002), in her account of those therapists who have been awarded a Fellowship by the College of Occupational Therapists, noted Constance Owens as the first occupational therapist to be awarded a PhD in 1962. The contributors of this book provide a range of examples of different career pathways. For therapists practising today, the rapidly emerging evidence base to practice, the development of new interventions, changing policy initiatives, the international dimension to practice and professional and regulatory requirements all demand active measures to keep up to date.

There are numerous ways to undertake continuing professional development, and Alsop (2000) describes over 90 methods, many of which are also recognised by the Health Professions Council (2005). Many of these activities would contribute to advancing practice, and keeping a reflective log, writing a book review, attending and presenting at conferences and participating in a journal club are clear examples.

While good practice and codes of conduct (College of Occupational Therapists, 2005 ; World Federation of Occupational Therapists, 2005) have always promoted continuing professional development, recent regulatory change in the UK (Health Professions Council, 2005) have added a degree of compulsion for individual therapists to record and provide confirmation of their achievements. While the exhortation to keep up with evidence in a current area of practice is sound, achieving it can be more challenging. This means more than just being aware of developments in occupational therapy and occupational science; it requires critical engagement with them.

At one time it may have been possible for therapists to remain current about the profession by reading their national occupational therapy journal. However, as occupational therapy has become more international and as therapists publish results of their research in other journals, this is no longer the case, as can be seen, for example, in the randomised controlled trial of community occupational therapy for people with dementia and their carers (Graff *et al.*, 2006). It is a sign of growing maturity that occupational therapy research is relevant in fields beyond the profession and it is also demonstrates the interprofessional nature of research. But therapists must also be aware of innovation in national and international policy and of advances in areas of practice that impact on the client groups with whom they work. Fortunately, along with the proliferation of literature, there has been an increase in the ease with which that literature can be accessed and utilised.

Further study

Although continuing professional development is more than just formal education, it is likely that becoming an advanced practitioner will involve some additional study. In the UK, the guidance on the development of consultant therapists suggested that these therapists should be educated to master's level (DH, 2000; Craik & McKay, 2003). Also in the UK, the revised grading structure for occupational therapists and other staff working in the NHS has suggested that promotion to grades requiring highly developed specialist knowledge and advanced theoretical knowledge will be linked with evidence of the attainment of qualifications at the master's and doctoral level (DH, 2004).

From a late start, occupational therapy education in the UK moved to an all-degree profession during the 1990s and there has also been an increase in the number of postgraduate and master's-level routes to qualification for those who have a primary degree in another subject. However, in North America, occupational therapy education has moved to all master's-level education as the pre-registration qualification, and it remains to be seen if that move will reach the UK. Such a development would certainly present challenges, as many other countries remain at diploma level or have just recently moved to degree-level education in occupational therapy.

While the requirement for occupational therapists to engage in continuing professional development and further study is great, so are the opportunities. With a first or second degree in occupational therapy, there are many routes to further study. Some of these will also be available to therapists with a diploma and confirmation of further study or experience. However, if the purpose is to advance practice in occupational therapy, then that further study must surely have an occupational focus. Fortunately, there are now many options for taught master's-level study. Until recently, further study has been seen as the route for senior practitioners usually with several years of post-qualification experience. Indeed, this has often been a prerequisite to obtaining funding for study. Often these therapists have studied part time, over 2 or 3 years, while coping with the demands of a senior post and family commitments, and it is to their credit that so many have achieved additional qualifications. While this career path will continue, other options are emerging, with a few therapists now embarking on further study, perhaps on a full-time basis, prior to a career in practice, academia or research.

In other academic disciplines, this would represent a standard career development pattern. Yet, in previous years when there was a shortage of therapists, further study on graduation was viewed as a controversial option. In current times, with a shortage of junior occupational therapy posts in the UK, this may be viewed differently. For some graduates, continuing study when they are in the frame of mind for academic work seems sensible, and mature students may feel that this assists in making up for their later start in an occupational therapy career. For other graduates, if an occupational therapy post is not immediately available, then engaging in further study, either at master's or doctoral level, may be a better option than accepting a less relevant job.

Doctoral studies and beyond

Although there has been an encouraging increase in the number of occupational therapists who have an MPhil or PhD throughout the world, there are still not enough and more must be done to encourage and support therapists to pursue this goal if the profession is to flourish. However, the acquisition of a research degree will have limited value to the profession if its focus is not firmly based in the realities of practice, and it will have limited value to service users if it does not establish original knowledge of relevance to improving their quality of life. Fortunately there are now more occupational therapists with the qualifications and experience to supervise research. This was not always the case, and many of the early therapists who embarked on research degree had to struggle to maintain an occupational focus in their study. Ironically, the anticipated reduction in posts for new graduates may be the catalyst to encourage some graduates to engage in full-time PhD studies. When jobs were plentiful, there was little incentive to study for a further 3 years on a limited PhD bursary; now for some graduates this may be an option. However, two therapists who pursued a PhD following their initial qualification later reported barriers in obtaining an occupational therapy post (Henderson & Maciver, 2003). Now, it is to be hoped that a more enlightened opinion would prevail. However, obtaining a PhD is only the first stage in a research career and more opportunities and funding must be created for postdoctoral research in collaboration with practice.

Research

The research theme is evident throughout this book and is the focus of several chapters. While the increase in occupational therapy research in recent years has been substantial, more is required if practice is to be advanced to benefit clients. If occupational therapists are not motivated to research their own practice, then other are unlikely to do so (Craik, 1997).

The transition of occupational therapy to degree-level education in some countries has been an important phase in ensuring that therapists have an appreciation of research and its influence on practice. However, there has sometimes been a naïve perception that, once this goal was attained, high-quality research would flow from these therapists. But as has been described, an all-degree profession is just the first stage in establishing a research culture in occupational therapy. In the UK, the College of Occupational Therapists, through its research and development strategies, suggested that, while all therapists should be consumers of research, 4.2 % of the occupational therapy graduates should be funded to ensure that sufficient therapists have PhDs and 1% of therapists would be expected to become research leaders (Illot & White, 2001). By 2007, these figures had not been achieved; however, the College continues to promote research and has ambitious plans to establish a UK Occupational Therapy Research Foundation (White & Creek, 2007). As with other disciplines, only when there is a critical mass of researchers, with a PhD or other research degree, who are engaged in funded full-time research, probably working in research teams, will high-quality research be produced.

This is not to devalue the research that has been, and is being, conducted. However, with some notable exceptions, much current published literature has not been completed as part of a funded study but as the result of individual study towards educational qualifications or from studies with little or limited funding. While these studies provide worthwhile information, they are frequently small scale, with few participants and sometimes not linked to other work. There is much debate within the profession about the relative merits of qualitative or quantitative methodologies and which provides the best quality of evidence to change practice. Perhaps a more pertinent debate should be how to facilitate the development of sufficient researchers and research teams capable of competing for research funds to move beyond the current positions. Returning to an optimistic perspective, there are some examples of this from other countries for example at the University of Southern California, where Florence Clark and colleagues work, (http://www.usc.edu/schools/ihp/ot/) and at the University of Illinois at Chicago, where Gary Kielhofner and colleagues are based (http://www.ahs.uic.edu/ot/).

Research practice collaborations

Continuing on a positive theme, there are encouraging developments in relation to establishing research practice collaborations, which are able to harness academics in university occupational therapy departments and practitioners to conduct research with larger numbers of clients. Lloyd et al. (2005) traced the progress of several of these in Australia from their inception through to the publication of results. However, they warned of the long-term commitment and funding that are required to produce worthwhile outcomes. In the United States, the Scholarship of Practice developments linked with the University of Illinois at Chicago provide an example that has been extended through UK Core (Forsyth et al., 2005). Other less formal partnerships have been created in the UK between academia and practice with some now reaching the stage of publication of outcome (Lim et al., 2007).

There is no universal template for a successful collaboration; rather, colleagues are encouraged to work with willing partners to create a symbiotic relationship that meets the needs and aspirations of all parties. However, the literature (Lloyd *et al.*, 2005) and experience (Craik & Morley, 2004; Craik & Watkeys, 2006) suggest that realistic time scales and dedicated funding are required to see these ventures move from ambition to achievement. Nevertheless, efforts in nurturing these collaborations between academic staff and practitioners can have many benefits especially for those with perseverance and patience. Initially they deliver the short-term outcome of a successful project, are able to advance practice in the clinical setting where it was conducted, and, through presentation and publication, bring these benefits to a larger audience. Further, they also construct a foundation for further study and they assist in building research teams that will be in a better position to apply for funding than an independent researcher.

With the possibility of some occupational therapy graduates being willing to undertake full-time PhD scholarship over 3 years, perhaps these research practice collaboration should investigate how to fund such scholarships, and certainly they need to develop the research questions to generate further studies. There is much to be done in replicating studies, linking smaller-scale studies together, conducting multi-site studies and exploring research opportunities with others. It is especially important to involve service users in this process to ensure the relevance of such research.

Catalysts to advance practice

Although it is the duty of individuals to maintain their professional competence and keep up-to-date with progress in evidence-based practice (College of Occupational Therapists, 2005; Health Professions Council, 2005), the organisations employing occupational therapists also have a responsibility to support them to do so. In the UK and elsewhere, this has led to the creation of a number of new therapy posts that may have different titles such as specialist practitioners, practice development posts and consultant therapists. Whatever the title, the concept of a therapist with a primary focus on advancing practice is useful and does not retract from the responsibility of others to do so; rather, it provides a catalyst to collective action within a service and the impetus to sustain and extend it. But in the current climate of financial constraints, it remains to be seen if these posts will continue to be funded. The evidence of their value can be seen in the pages of this book, with several chapters written by holders of these posts.

However, even in services where no such posts exist and no additional funding is available, imaginative occupational therapy managers can find ways to obtain the same effect. Occupational therapists are creative and optimistic people; they could not be effective therapists without these attributes. The history of the profession, especially in mental health, has been carved by therapists who have a vision of how service could be and have made it happen.

This can be achieved by examining the policy directives or mission statement of a service and finding the potential link with occupational therapy. There is seldom any point in searching the index of a new policy document for the words 'occupational therapy'; they are unlikely to be there unless an occupational therapist was a member of the policy group. It is more effective to seek key words for their relevance. Ormston (1999) pointed out that the UK's research priorities (DH, 1999, p. 116) included 'developing and evaluating a range of occupational activities to maximise social participation, enhance self-esteem and improve clinical outcomes'. A clearer call to occupational therapy would be hard to find. In the UK, recent policy on social inclusion (Office of the Deputy Prime Minister, 2004) and on vocational rehabilitation (Department of Work and Pensions, 2004) have led to an increased focus on these areas. Internationally, the World Health Organisation's (2001) publication of the *International Classification of Functioning, Disability and Health* provided an opportunity to consider these issues from an occupational perspective, and the College of Occupational Therapists (2004) published guidance on how to link this to health promotion. Thus, the creative occupational therapy manager can find ways to meet the needs of the organisation and advance practice to the benefit of service users.

New directions for occupational therapy

It is always difficult to decide what direction to pursue, with only the past and present as a guide. However, the rapid growth of occupational therapy in forensic mental health over the past 15 years is an interesting example. The recent suggestion that the UK will establish new specialist units for mentally ill prisoners with an emphasis on rehabilitation would create an opportunity for the expansion of the current limited presence of occupational therapy in the prison service. Thus, the knowledge and skills that occupational therapists have acquired in forensic mental health could be transferred into a related and developing area of practice.

The UK appears to be at the end of a period of unprecedented growth in the profession in terms of numbers of therapists, students and influence. But that growth has been accompanied by penalties. The impetus for the expansion has come from the NHS with the consequent constraints that large organisations impose; so in some respects it could be viewed as stifling progress in other sectors. Practice in other counties has a more diverse base, and different opportunities may now be more open to UK therapists. There are excellent models from other countries to provide guidance, for example, the emphasis on vocational rehabilitation from Canada and Australia. This further emphasises the international aspects of modern occupational therapy and the need to read international literature and seek examples from other countries.

Developing these new opportunities will involve working beyond traditional and statutory services, but there is often more freedom in voluntary organisations to pursue the objectives that are at the heart of the profession. So, these new directions may actually involve the profession returning to its roots, which may be to everyone's advantage. In moving forward to meet the challenges of the future, it will be important to retain the best of occupational therapy of the past but not to be afraid to leave behind those practices that do not have an evidence base and are not to true to principles of the founders of the profession. With the current emphasis on work–life balance, well-being, health promotion and the growth of jobs with titles such as life coach, there are clear associations with traditional occupational therapy territory. There is an intriguing world out there beckoning us, if we have the courage and imagination to take advantage of the opportunities.

So, is the future optimistic or pessimistic? Do we have sufficient therapists with the vision and passion to make the best of what we have and not lament what we do not? My career has been based on the belief that we do. Will you take up the challenge and make this happen?

Questioning your Practice

1. What is your personal action plan to advance your own practice over the next 3 years?
2. How do you plan to advance the practice of the team or service you work with?
3. What will your contribution be to advancing the profession?

References

Alsop A (2000) *Continuing Professional Development: A Guide for Therapists.* Oxford: Blackwell Science.

College of Occupational Therapists (2004) *College of Occupational Therapists' Guidance on the use of The International Classification of Functioning, Disability and Health (ICF) and the Ottawa Charter for Health Promotion in Occupational Therapy Services.* London: College of Occupational Therapists.

College of Occupational Therapists (2005) *Code of Ethics and Professional Conduct for Occupational Therapists.* London: College of Occupational Therapists.

Craik C (1997) Research: Moving from Debate to Action. *British Journal of Occupational Therapy, 60(2),* 65–66.

Craik C, Austin C, Chacksfield J D, *et al.* (1998) College of Occupational Therapists: position paper on the way ahead for research, education and practice in mental health. *British Journal of Occupational Therapy, 61(9),* 390–392.

Craik C, McKay E (2003) Consultant therapists: recognising and developing expertise. *British Journal of Occupational Therapy, 66(6),* 281–283.

Craik C, Morley M (2004) Building research into mental health practice. Poster presented at 23rd September 2006 the European Occupational Therapy Conference, Athens, Greece.

Craik C, Pieris Y (2006) Without leisure … 'it wouldn't be much of a life': the meaning of leisure for people with mental health problems living in the community. *British Journal of Occupational Therapy, 69(5),* 209–216.

Craik C, Watkeys F (2006) Sustaining research collaborations in forensic mental health occupational therapy. Poster presented at the *25th July 2006 International Congress of World Federation of Occupational Therapists*, Sydney, Australia.

Department of Health (1999) National Service Framework for Mental Health. http://www.dh.gov. uk/assetRoot/04/07/72/09/04077209.pdf (accessed 26 March 2007).

Department of Health (2000) *Meeting the Challenge: A Strategy for the Allied Health Professions.* London: HMSO.

Department of Health (2004) *NHS Job Evaluation Handbook* (2nd Edn). http://www.dh.gov.uk/ en/Publicationsandstatistics/Publications/PublicationsPolicyAndGuidance/DH_4090845.(accessed 26 March 2007).

Department of Work and Pensions (2004) Building capacity for work: A UK framework for vocational rehabilitation. http://www.dwp.gov.uk/publications/vrframework/dwp_vocational_rehabilitation. pdf (accessed 26 March 2007).

Farndale J (1961) *The Day Hospital Movement in Great Britain.* Oxford: Pergamon Press.

Forsyth K, Summerfield Mann L, Kielhofner G (2005) Scholarship of practice: making occupation-focused, theory-driven, evidence-based practice a reality. *British Journal of Occupational Therapy, 68(6),* 260–268.

Graff MJL, Vernooij-Dassen MJM, Thijssen M, *et al.* (2006) Community based occupational therapy for patients with dementia and their care givers: randomised controlled trial. *British Medical Journal,* http://www.bmj.com/cgi/content/full/333/7580/1196. Accessed 26 March 2007. DOI:10.1136/bmj. 39001.688843.BE.

Health Professions Council (2005) Continuing professional development and your registration. http:// www.hpc-uk.org/assets/documents/10001314CPD_and_your_registration.pdf (accessed 1 March 2007).

Henderson SE, Maciver D (2003) To PhD or not to PhD: the question is, where we work? *British Journal of Occupational Therapy, 66(10),* 482–484.

Illot I, White E (2001) 2001 College of Occupational Therapists' research and development strategic vision and action plan. *British Journal of Occupational Therapy, 64(6),* 270–277.

Lim KH, Morris J, Craik C (2007) Inpatients' perspectives of occupational therapy in acute mental health. *Australian Occupational Therapy Journal, (54),* 22–32.

Lloyd C, King R, Bassett H (2005) Occupational therapy and clinical research in mental health rehabilitation. *British Journal of Occupational Therapy, 68(4),* 172–176.

Office of the Deputy Prime Minister (2004). *Mental Health and Social Exclusion. Social Exclusion Unit Report Summary.* London: HMSO.

Ormston C (1999) The national service framework for mental health: worth waiting for? *Occupational Therapy News,* December 10–12.

White E, Creek J (2007) College of Occupational Therapists' research and development strategic vision and action plan: 5 year review. *British Journal of Occupational Therapy, 70(3),* 122–128.

Wilcock AA (2002) *Occupation for Health; A Journey from Prescription to Self Health.* London: College of Occupational Therapists.

World Federation of Occupational Therapists (2005) Code of ethics. http://www.wfot.org.au/office_ files/WFOTCode%20of%20Ethics%202005.pdf (accessed 20 March 2007).

World Health Organisation (2001) *International Classification of Functioning, Disability and Health.* Geneva: World Health Organisation.

Index